Natural Health and Wellness Encyclopedia

By John Waldrop
and
Janice McCall Failes

Acknowledgments

To June Gunden, whose skills as an editor are unsurpassed.

To Alice Johnston, for your conscientiousness and hard work in typesetting the manuscript.

To Debbie Williams, for your artwork and design.

To all the staff of FC&A for your support and help and, especially, thanks and praise to our Lord and Savior, Jesus Christ, who gives us strength and the promise of eternal life.

Pleasant words are like a honeycomb,

Sweetness to the soul and health to the body.

—PROVERBS 16:24

For I will restore health to you,

And your wounds will I heal,

Says the Lord

—JEREMIAH 30:17a

Table of Contents

Introduction

Natural Health and Wellness Encyclopedia is a treasure house of all the latest information about what you can do to improve your health. It tells you how to help prevent or relieve many health problems. It has been written simply to explain some of the fascinating tips that easily can be used for a naturally healthier life.

Many of the suggestions reported may be controversial or unproven by controlled scientific studies. We have reported the ideas in this book because there is some evidence that they have worked for some people. In doing this, we have attempted to separate fact from fiction and to give special attention to health tips which have been confirmed by scientific research. We have attempted, wherever possible, to verify the accuracy of information reported in this book. Nevertheless, since these are reports of the research or ideas of other people, we cannot guarantee their safety or effectiveness.

Because of the possibility of errors in reporting, and because medical science is such a rapidly expanding field with new developments reported each day, we ask that you consult carefully with your own physician before trying any of the ideas listed in this book.

The health tips reported in this book are not guaranteed to succeed with everyone. As we wrote this book, we realized that we could not pass judgment on the effectiveness of all of the health tips that we discovered. Some of these tips may work for you but not for other people. Some may work for others but not for you.

It can be dangerous to rely on self-treatment or home remedies and neglect proven medical treatments, such as surgery in cases of cancer. Medical treatment shouldn't be ignored, but natural prevention or treatment may help, too. A good physician is the best judge of what sort of medical treatment may be needed for certain diseases. It's good to choose a doctor who is open-minded about safe, natural methods of healing.

Best wishes as you strive for a naturally healthier life. We believe this book will help you.

AGE SPOTS

A Nutrient That Helps Prevent Age Spots

Are those dark purple spots that appear in old age inevitable? No, according to Dr. Oscar Gyde, a British hematologist.

A test of 20 elderly patients with age spots and 20 without at England's Fast Birmingham Hospital revealed that besides the age spots "the only measurable difference between the two groups was the level of zinc in their body," Gyde says. "The elderly without the spots on their skin had a higher level of zinc. The elderly with spots had a significantly lower level of zinc," says Gyde.

Dr. Gyde concluded from the study that age spots "are not simply an unsightly sign of aging. Their presence means you should suspect a zinc deficiency."

The purple spots, not to be confused with brown age spots which are freckles that have spread, occur when the tiny blood vessels in the skin rupture and bleed. They eventually disappear on their own, Gyde explains.

"The role of zinc would be to prevent them from appearing in the first place or from reappearing," he says.

Dr. Mary Dundas of the University of Tennessee advises eating foods high in zinc as a preventative. Those foods include such high protein fares as shellfish, oysters, red meat and liver.

You may also want to check with your doctor about zinc supplements, Dr. Gyde adds. The recommended daily dietary allowance of zinc for adults is 15 mg. per day.

A Procedure That Makes Age Spots Disappear

Many elderly people who are otherwise attractive and healthy wish that somehow they could get rid of those telltale age spots and freckles.

Now there's hope. With the use of a new laser, blemishes can be removed without a noticeable scar, reports Dr. Bruce Smoller of Harvard Medical School. The low-dose carbon dioxide laser will remove the age spots and freckles painlessly, and the procedure is so quick that it can be done in a walk-in clinic.

One word of caution: Any unusual change in a mole or blemish should be reported to your doctor.

AGING PROBLEMS

A Natural Wellspring of Wellness

Since the creation of the world water has been known as a source of life. It is still one of the best secrets to overall health.

This is especially true as we age. Yet, many elderly people lose their sense of thirst, reports the *New England Journal of Medicine.* According to the study, older people must be particularly careful to drink eight glasses of water each day even though they may not feel thirsty or uncomfortable.

Water helps your body in many ways. It is necessary for regular bowel movements, it helps prevent kidney stones, it protects the body against disease, and it helps to regulate body temperature. In addition, drinking lots of water will avoid high concentrations of prescription drugs in the kidneys and prevent dehydration.

It is remarkable that so many benefits can come from so inexpensive and plentiful a source. Here's to your health!

ALCOHOL PROBLEMS

This Vitamin Helps
Neutralize Effects of Alcohol

Orange juice may not be your drink of choice at cocktail parties. But if researchers at the University of Michigan had their way, a tall pitcher of O.J. would be mandatory at every party.

The Michigan researchers studied college students to determine the effect of vitamin C on blood alcohol levels, *Prevention* magazine reports. When the students were put on a "laboratory-controlled drinking spree," alcohol was cleared from their blood faster after having taken "5,000 milligrams of time-release vitamin C for two weeks."

Vincent G. Zannoni, Ph.D., and Robert Susick Jr., Ph.D., who conducted the study, say the faster alcohol clears from your blood stream, the faster you sober up and the less chance you have of contracting liver disease.

They found vitamin C actually blunted the effects of drunkenness. Although counting backwards by sevens was no easier for those who had taken vitamin C supplements, the students could bring their finger tips together better and distinguish between subtle colors.

Based on the study, Dr. Zannoni thinks "vitamin C can help protect the average drinker from some of the consequences of alcohol consumption." Still, the best safeguard is to drink in moderation. As Zannoni says: "Everyone should probably drink a little less, and get a little more vitamin C."

A Common Mistake

Many people who have overindulged in alcohol seek relief from their discomfort by reaching for that familiar bottle of aspirin. What's wrong with that?

The fact is that if you take plain aspirin to treat your hangover you may be asking for a new problem. It is not uncommon for aspirin to cause stomach irritation.

It's better to take coated aspirin (often called enteric-coated aspirin) because it will not be released in the stomach.

Buffered aspirin or acetaminophen (like Tylenol®) will also cause fewer stomach problems while still calming the hangover.

ALLERGIES

Attacking That Airborne Allergy

Before you despair of ever breathing freely again, why not launch an attack on that allergy? The best offense, we know, is a good defense. So the first step is to learn what to avoid that might be causing your allergy.

Here are some common allergens (things that trigger allergic symptons):

- dust and molds
- animal hair or feathers
- strong odors
- petroleum-based gases and fumes or dust associated with coal heat
- insecticides
- hair sprays
- perfumes
- waxes and polishes
- detergents and bleach
- room deodorizers
- gasoline
- paint and paint thinners
- tar
- plastics
- lubricants

- asphalt and cement
- cigarette, cigar and pipe smoke
- inhaled insect parts. Hairs, scales or other body parts of insects like houseflies, mayflies, moths, cockroaches, spiders, honeybees, caddis flies, locusts and mites may cause problems.
- pollen.

Sneezing, runny nose, nasal congestion, shortness of breath, sore throat, watery eyes, itchy eyes or wheezing are the most common allergic reactions to airborne particles.

The best way to relieve allergy symptoms is to avoid the allergen if it is known. To guard against aggravating your allergy to airborne things:

- Mow the lawn regularly to help lower grass pollen.
- Cut all weeds as soon as possible.
- Use air-conditioning in your house. Central air-conditioning helps control airborne allergens. A window air-conditioner is recommended for the bedroom of the allergy sufferer.
- Use air filters (electrostatic air filters if possible).
- Change vacuum cleaner filters. A central vacuum cleaning system is best because the system won't exhaust air and dust into the living area. If

you don't have a central system, be sure to keep the windows open when vacuuming.

• Radiant heat is best for allergy sufferers. Forced air heat circulates dust and causes the house to dry out.

• Keep your office and home as clean as possible, especially bedrooms.

• Avoid housecleaning while the allergy suffering person is present.

• Use non-allergenic covers on mattresses and pillows.

• Use polyester or other non-allergenic pillows, and replace them at least every three years.

• Vacuum fabric-covered furniture frequently.

• Don't keep houseplants that have a strong fragrance or plants that require a lot of water because they could mildew.

• Use an artificial Christmas tree to reduce the possibility of mold and mildew.

• Have washable curtains and avoid heavy draperies.

• Don't hang wet clothes or linens outside to dry. Use a dryer and keep the filter clean.

• Don't use rugs, carpets, stuffed toys, furry toys, quilts or afghans in the bedroom.

• Don't use strong-smelling cleaners, polishes, moth balls, perfume or chemicals in the bedroom.

- Don't use aerosol sprays of any kind.
- Store books in boxes or warm, dry areas. Get rid of old books which may have mildewed.
- Sterilize the air ducts at the beginning of each cold season. Clean the air ducts and filters regularly.
- Keep household pets out of bedrooms or out of the house if possible.
- Don't allow cigarettes, pipes or cigars to be smoked in or around the house.
- Avoid using wallpaper in the bedrooms.
- Keep physically fit and exercise regularly. Congestion in the nose may be worse when you are resting or sitting still than when you are active. Exercise can be as simple as swimming, walking or bike riding. Exercising indoors may protect you from allergens in the outside air.
- Maintain good general health.
- Avoid breathing fine powders like talcum powder, dusting powder or powdered artificial sweeteners like Equal® or Sweet 'N Low®. They can irritate the breathing system.
- Keep the windows and vents of your car closed when driving. Use air-conditioning in your car.
- Avoid early morning activity. According to the American Academy of Allergies, pollen is

heaviest in the air before 10:00 a.m.

• Avoid extreme temperature changes. Follow the weather forecast so you can avoid strong winds, drastic changes in humidity, barometric pressure or temperature.

• Asthmatics and people with allergies to airborne particles should stay indoors for a day after a heavy storm. A report in the medical journal *Lancet* (1:1079) says that fungus spores and small particles of pollen may stay in the air after a large storm.

• Consider taking a long vacation. Sometimes a long vacation is enough to help relieve severe allergic reactions. Plan your vacation during the peak of the season when your allergy flares up. If possible, go where you won't be affected by your allergen.

• If you must live in a big city, try to avoid congested areas with heavy traffic because cars and trucks create noxious exhaust fumes. Avoid areas with known industrial pollution.

But I've Never
Been Allergic To
That Before!

People often wonder why they suddenly react to a product that they have been using for several years, perhaps throughout their whole lives. But many times people reach a sensitivity point—that means that the body may be able to tolerate the allergen in small doses, but the body eventually reaches its tolerance level, and an allergic reaction occurs.

Some women discover allergies while they are pregnant. Many of these allergies will disappear after the birth of the child. However, some women with severe allergies have experienced the opposite effect—their allergies have cleared up during their pregnancies!

Some people suffer from an allergy for the first time after a move to a new area. If you've had severe allergies in the past and are considering a move to a different area, be careful to take an extended visit there before making a complete move. Some areas may be great for certain allergy sufferers but not for you. Many allergy sufferers will develop a new allergy once they have lived in a community for a while. Do not rush into a permanent move.

Allergy-sensitive people need to be detectives and learn everything that causes them to react, the *Lancet* journal (1:617) suggests.

Cockroaches Cause Allergies

Cockroaches are unsightly pests. They elicit many negative reactions: screaming, fainting, throwing of objects, sneezing. Sneezing?

That's right. What some people believe to be a reaction to household dust may really be an allergic response to cockroaches. Cockroaches were found to cause allergic reactions in one hundred New Orleans allergy sufferers, according to *The Journal of Allergy and Clinical Immunology*.

Live American and German roaches were frozen, dipped in physiologic salines and "mixed" in a blender for five minutes. The mixture was then stirred, sterile filtered and stored at low temperatures.

The subjects were skin pricked with the cockroach whole body extracts and extracts of common allergens (things that cause allergies). Forty-eight percent of those who reacted to at least two of the common allergens reacted immediately to the cockroach extract. The study established for the first time that cockroaches are a source of significant allergens.

More than half the subjects had asthma, "which may in part be exerbated by cockroach exposure," the *Journal* says. Other studies have confirmed that opinion.

You might be trying to deal with a house dust allergy when cockroaches are the real culprit. The two allergies do not go hand in hand. The New Orleans study found that 25 percent of the subjects who had positive reactions to American cockroach extract had no reaction to house dust.

Cosmetics As a Cause of Allergies

Cosmetics include make-up and the many products both sexes use to clean, condition and "beautify" their hair and bodies. Allergic reactions are quite common to the following cosmetics: deodorants, soap, perfume, cologne, shaving cream, after-shave lotion, shampoo, mouthwash, lipstick, eyeliner, mascara, eye shadow, blush, foundation, hair dye, hair bleach, hair coloring, hair spray, hair mousse, skin cleanser, hair remover, suntan lotion, tanning cream, nail polish, nail polish remover and the glue on artificial nails.

Localized allergic reactions to these products may cause skin rash, dryness or irritation. General allergic reactics can affect the whole body by causing hives, congestion, asthma or swelling. Many allergic reactions to cosmetics can cause premature aging of the skin if it becomes damaged. The most commonly occurring reaction to cosmetics is skin dermatitis, with symptoms like irritation, redness, itching, swelling, rash, scaling, blisters and dryness.

The best method of treating cosmetic allergies is to avoid the offending cosmetics. However, until you know which cosmetics are causing the problem, here are some suggestions to help keep the reactions from becoming unbearable:

• Keep your body, hair and clothes as clean as possible. Avoid touching your face or eyes with your hands. For example, if you rub your eyes, your hand lotion may irritate them.

• If you think you know what product you are allergic to, try switching to a different brand. Sometimes the allergen may be an ingredient that only one manufacturer uses. However, changing products is recommended only if the initial allergic reaction was not severe.

• Consider and evaluate the ingredients before purchasing a cosmetic product. Unfortunately, to protect secret formulas, federal regulations allow some ingredients to be listed in very general categories. This may make it difficult to determine if the cosmetic you select contains the offending allergen.

• Try switching to hypoallergenic cosmetics.

However, according to the Allergy Foundation of America, not all hypoallergenic cosmetics meet their manufacturer's claims.

• If you discover that you can use certain cosmetics, try to keep your applicators very clean. Your allergies may be a reaction to make-up applicators like sponges, brushes, eye wands and puffs. Keeping them very clean or trying new ways to apply your make-up may help relieve the allergy.

• If truly hypoallergenic products don't eliminate the reactions, stop using all make-up and cosmetics. After about six months of being completely allergy-free, you can try reintroducing some cosmetics one at a time if your reactions were not too serious or life-threatening. You may discover that you can use some products but not others.

• Use a bland, unscented soap to wash your face, skin and hair. Using the soap on your hair will help wash away any remains of your previous shampoo and conditioner.

• Try to stop using any lotions or creams like hand lotion, baby oil, cleansing cream or moisturizers. When showering or bathing, use warm water, not hot. Hot water dries out your skin, making it more sensitive.

• Avoid using nail polish. Nail polish can cause allergic reactions in many places, not just on your hands. Nail polish can irritate eyes or facial skin, since we touch our eyes and face with our fingers and hands. Even a man can experience an allergic reaction to a woman's nail polish or other cosmetics if he is in close contact with her!

• Discuss your allergies and concerns with your hairdresser. You may discover that one of the hair products is causing your allergic reaction. If the hairdresser doesn't have alternative products or won't serve you with little or no cosmetics, find another beauty or barber shop. Also, if you plan to have your hair tinted, colored or permed, insist on a skin test before the full treatment. A small skin test and a little patience can prevent a severe reaction later.

Is It an Allergy? Or Just a Reaction To Your Prescription?

If you have developed congestion, hives, swelling, skin rashes and dryness, or asthma, you may be searching frantically for the cause of what you think is an "allergic reaction."

But wait. If you are taking a prescription drug, check with your doctor to make sure the reaction is not a known side effect or a photosensitive reaction to your medicine. Photosensitive reactions occur when you're exposed to sunlight while taking a prescribed drug.

Perhaps a change in medication will be all you need to get relief.

Seasonal Allergies—Sneezing by the Calendar

Many people have seasonal allergies, like an allergy to pollen or mold. Some of these allergies are nicknamed "hay fever," but the name is not accurate. It isn't hay, but pollen, that causes the problem, and the problem isn't a fever but an allergic reaction!

The pollen season begins in February in the southern United States, but starts later the farther north you travel. "Pollen counts," which measure the amount of pollen in the air in a 24-hour period, are available on many TV weather programs to help you. According to the American Academy of Allergy and Immunology, a count of 50 or more is considered high, 30-50 is moderate, and 10-20 is a low count. During the heavy pollen season in your area, or a day with a high pollen count, you should avoid going outside or opening your windows.

Be aware of which seasons of the year are the

times when your allergy flares up, and take special precautions during those times.

The Hidden Danger
of Nasal Sprays

Congestion, stuffy nose, breathing problems—all can be helped by using a nasal spray. But that same nasal spray, used improperly, can actually increase your allergic symptoms, according to the Food and Drug Administration (FDA).

If you don't follow the package instructions on over-the-counter nasal sprays, you may suffer from a "rebound" effect and the spray may begin to cause swelling in the nasal tissues. Nasal sprays are supposed to be used for only short term relief—three days at the most. But many allergy sufferers try to rely on the spray throughout the allergy season. Overuse of sprays can also lead to side effects like drowsiness, an increased heart rate, nervousness, burning, and sneezing.

When used properly the sprays are helpful but many people abuse them, the FDA reports. For best relief:

- never use a spray for more than three days
- never use more than the package recommends
- never lean back when applying the spray

• never share the spray with anyone else—it is unsanitary.

Allergic to Your
Chewing Gum?

Food and food additives are known to trigger allergies, but it is often difficult to track down the additives in everything we eat.

A sudden inflammation of the blood vessels can be caused by the additive BHT (butylated hydroxytoluene), found in some chewing gum. BHT is a perservative added to many products like salted peanuts, cake mixes, potato chips and chewing gum. If you develop a sudden skin rash or allergic reaction, be sure to consider all the products you have been eating or using.

For an interesting study on the relation of food allergies to arthritis pain, see the article "Relieve Arthritis Pain by Avoiding Certain Foods?"

ALZHEIMER'S DISEASE

A Vitamin That
May Help

Alzheimer's disease is a senile deterioration of the mind which usually results in death within a few months or years after the first symptoms become evident. Memory loss is one of the chief symptoms of Alzheimer's disease, but an accurate diagnosis should be made by a competent physician, since some memory loss is normal as people age.

No one knows the cause of Alzheimer's disease. Some physicians suspect a slow-acting virus or viral particle which attacks the brain. Others think an autoimmune reaction to antigens in cigarette smoke may be one cause of the disease, because smokers are four times more likely to get the disease than non-smokers.

There is no cure for Alzheimer's disease, but the vitamin choline is reported in one study to slightly slow down the irreversible brain deterioration or at least to improve memory somewhat in the sufferers of this disease.

This Food May Help Prevent
Alzheimer's Disease

Autopsies of Alzheimer victims have revealed higher than normal levels of aluminum in the brain tissue. Aluminum can get into the body from drinking water, baking powder, flour and cake mixes, pancake mixes, table salt, salad dressings, frozen dough, self-rising flour, processed cheese, some pickled cucumbers, nondairy creamers, buffered aspirin, antacids, anti-diarrhea products, douches, aluminum pots and pans, deodorants, skin creams, lipsticks, lotions, and hemorrhoid creams.

Theoretically, preventing the accumulation of aluminum in elderly people may slow or prevent the development of the disease, but scientific studies haven't been completed to prove or disprove this theory. According to some researchers these three things may help prevent the accumulation of aluminum in the brains of Alzheimer victims:

- avoiding foods containing aluminum,
- drinking three glasses of skim milk per day,
- taking fluoride supplements.

Alzheimer's Disease?
Or Is It a Simple
Vitamin Deficiency?

One of the most heart-breaking diagnoses an elderly person can get is: "You have Alzheimer's disease."

But some of these diagnoses are wrong, according to *American Family Physician* (36,5:196). A lack of vitamin B12 (cobalamin) causes symptoms that could be mistaken for Alzheimer's disease. Depression, confusion, loss of reflexes, difficulty in walking and numbness of the feet are signs of vitamin B12 deficiency.

Since the absorption of B12 decreases with age, it is important that older people make sure they get adequate B12 in their diet or through supplements. The Recommended Dietary Allowance (RDA) for adults is 3.0 micrograms of cobalamin daily. Natural sources include liver, meat, milk, dairy products, fish and eggs.

It has also been found that intestinal diseases or long-term use of aspirin, acetaminophen, codeine, oral contraceptives or neomycin can interfere with the body's absorption of vitamin B12 and cause a deficiency. People diagnosed as having Alzheimer's disease may want to try B12 supplements. Maybe they have been wrongly diagnosed!

Alzheimer's Patients Can Improve Their Memory

Where were you when Kennedy was shot? When the space shuttle Challenger exploded? Many people not only remember where they were at those times, but they recall all sorts of details unrelated to the incident like what they wore or what they said.

It had been thought that such events "stimulated neurochemical activity that resulted in stronger memory," *Psychology Today* explains. But the article adds that psychologist Curt Sandman sought another explanation through an experiment with a new memory-enhancing technique. What he discovered could help improve memories of everyone from Alzheimer patients to those just getting forgetful in old age.

The traditional medical approach to memory loss encourages patients to establish and maintain routines, but Sandman encouraged his patients to seek variety.

The first test involved thirteen patients with Alzheimer's disease who had severe memory disorders. Sandman had them plan and carry out with their spouses a significant event each week and discuss it with them. The events included everything from buying new tires to going on a picnic in which exotic fruits were selected and eaten.

Ten of the thirteen patients showed striking improvement after two to five days. They recalled the day of the event four or five times better than they could a typical day and often they remembered it as clearly as their spouses did.

The technique was almost as therapeutic to the spouses as to the patients Sandman says, because they received a much-needed boost. The event was usually the couple's first positive shared experience in months or years.

Further trials confirmed the results. The patients sometimes recalled almost perfectly the things that happened on the day of the significant event, while on the afternoon of an eventless day they could not even remember what they ate for breakfast. The researchers will now try to extend the memory-enhanced period, and to help the patients make the connections required.

The experiments are significant for all of us as we get older. Much age-related memory loss can be warded off by engaging in different and fun activities, Sandman concludes.

ARTHRITIS

Relieve Arthritis Pain
By Avoiding Certain Foods?

The role of nutrition on arthritis has been observed and discussed for many years. Yet doctors have consistently refused to look at the possibility that food allergies may cause or worsen arthritis, according to *Prevention* magazine.

However the article goes on to cite a report in *Rheumatology News* which finally concedes that eating certain foods can worsen rheumatoid arthritis. Avoiding those foods can produce complete remission from the disease in some patients.

Thirty-one arthritis patients were tested to determine their reactions to certain foods, and the average patient reacted to about seven. Cereal grains were the biggest offender, with red meats running second. Reaction to vegetables and fruits were generally pretty low.

More than half of those tested for reactions to food additives and contaminants developed symptoms and four were so badly affected they couldn't complete the study. The researchers found that arthritis symptoms of several patients disappeared as long as they stayed away from the offending food.

The study also supported to some degree the belief that "nightshade" foods like tomatoes, potatoes, eggplant and peppers, will intensify symptoms.

Some people are sensitive to nightshade foods. One group has allergic reactions. Another larger group has toxic responses. For those patients, a single indulgence can trigger arthritic pain and swelling, even after months of abstinence from the nightshade. Withdrawal from an allergen for a long time, on the other hand, ordinarily eliminates allergic reactions.

Control This Culprit of Arthritis Pain

Reduce the salt in your diet if you suffer from arthritis, says Floyd Pennington, PhD., of the Arthritis Foundation, National Office in Atlanta. Since salt (sodium) causes swelling and water retention, it may cause additional stress on joints and increase the arthritis pain and problems. Pennington recommends a low salt diet which is better for your blood pressure as well as helping reduce arthritis symptoms.

If you are taking Ifen®, Motrin®, or Rufen® for the pain of arthritis, it may interfere with blood pressure medication.

An Unfriendly Carrier

You have always known that tick bites are a nuisance, but did you know they can cause arthritis?

One type of arthritis, known as Lyme arthritis, is spread by woodticks. The disease was named after Lyme, Connecticut, where it was first discovered.

A bacterium that causes arthritis symptoms is spread through the tick bites, according to *Science* magazine. Most people notice the bite and then a gradual thickening of the skin around the bite. Then, weeks or even months later, the bite victims start experiencing heat, pain, redness and swelling, usually in the large joints.

Pain relievers can be used to treat Lyme arthritis, but a doctor should be contacted immediately if this type of arthritis is suspected, since heart and brain problems can also be caused by this infection. Prompt medical attention will help reduce the amount of permanent damage to the joints, heart or brain.

ASTHMA

Some Little-Known Causes
of Asthma Attacks

Finding the substances that cause an asthmatic attack can be very difficult because many asthmatics react to different irritants.

The American Lung Association says that food odors can be bothersome to asthmatics. Strong odors are inhaled into the lungs and can start a bout of asthma. Asthmatics need to be aware of all their senses as they seek to overcome their disease.

Shane McDermott of the American Lung Association reveals that about 20 percent of asthmatic adults are bothered by aspirin. Aspirin is often overlooked as an asthma irritant, but it does trigger attacks. Monitor your reactions to all substances carefully and work with your doctor to keep your asthma under control, McDermott suggests.

Asthmatic? This Food Seasoning
Can Be Dangerous!

A high salt intake may increase the risk of death in asthmatics, especially in males, a study from

Great Britain reports. The risk of death increased by 40 percent in asthmatic men with a high salt intake, Dr. Peter Burney of London, England, discovered. But the highest risk seems to be in asthmatic children. A high salt diet could increase their chances of death by as much as three hundred percent! However, salt intake didn't seem to effect the death rate in women with asthma.

Dr. Burney recommends that all asthmatics cut back on salt and discuss diet with their doctors.

Some Prescription Drugs That May Help Asthmatics

A prescription drug used to treat ulcers may help reduce asthma in some patients, reports the *Archives of Internal Medicine* (147:56). Researchers found that patients who suffered from asthma and heartburn had fewer asthma attacks while taking Zantac® (ranitidine). However, when treatment with Zantac® ceased, their breathing became more difficult. It seems that the reflex which causes the heartburn also bothers the respiratory system and causes an asthmatic attack. Although Zantac® will not help all asthmatics, the researchers suggest that those who also suffer from chronic heartburn may be helped, as well as people whose asthma is worst when they are lying down.

An anti-cancer medicine may help some severe asthmatics, states the *New England Journal of Medicine* (318:10, 603). In severe cases of asthma, people often require daily doses of steroids like prednisone to help regulate breathing. However, prednisone (Deltasone®) has some strong side effects like fluid retention, muscle weakness, ulcers, increased perspiration, dizziness, headaches, blood-sugar problems, glaucoma, sleeplessness, and a decreased resistance to infections.

Now doctors are experimenting with the drug methotrexate, normally used to treat cancer, used in combination with steroids. So far, the studies have shown that asthmatics can cut back and perhaps even eliminate steroids (and those side effects) as long as they're taking methotrexate.

BACK PROBLEMS

New Alternative to Back Surgery

There were almost half a million operations for spinal disk problems in a recent year, according to *Prevention* magazine. The most famous disk problem that year, however, was not operated on— at least not in the traditional way.

When Joe Montana, the quarterback of the San Francisco Forty-Niners, went down with a ruptured disk, few thought he would play again that season. Some considered his career finished.

A procedure called "suction diskectomy," however, allowed him to return to action in time to lead his team into the play-offs.

The new treatment involves use of a "needlelike probe to cut away the protruding disk material and remove it by suction," *Prevention* reports.

Dr. Vert Mooney, chairman of the division of orthopedic surgery at the University of Texas Health Science Center, cites the procedure's advantages over conventional surgery: "It's done under local anesthesia, the amount of surrounding tissue destruction is minimal, and it's less invasive," he says.

The hospital stay for traditional surgery may be

as long as a week. A diskectomy, on the other hand, can be performed in the morning and the patient can leave by the end of the day, Mooney says.

Mooney adds that because conventional surgery is more involved, complications sometimes arise, leaving many patients with recurring pain. Only in extreme cases has the new procedure not been as effective as the old.

Natural Ways to Fight Back Pain

Excruciating back pain must be caused by a serious injury, right? Wrong. Most back pain can be avoided or greatly reduced by altering the way we move every day.

Here are some tips to help you prevent this troublesome malady:

• Avoid moving suddenly. Sharp or sudden movements can aggravate back pain. Getting out of a car too quickly after sitting still for a long time or jumping up to answer the phone can be very dangerous for back problems. Learn to move slowly and carefully.

• Straining your neck muscles can aggravate your back. Don't hold the phone between your neck and your ear, even with a phone rest. Always hold the phone with your hand to avoid tensing up the neck muscles.

• Be careful when doing housework. We often underestimate how difficult housework is. Be sure to take breaks between doing heavy tasks. Stretch your back and neck muscles, as you would before exercising. By stretching them before the heavy tasks you will help prepare them and could avoid unnecessary muscle strain.

• Push, don't pull. Pulling heavy objects creates more strain on your lower back than pushing the object. If you suffer from back problems, don't be afraid to ask for help to move large objects.

• Move around frequently. Don't stay in one position for a long period of time. If you are driving, flying in an airplane, or working at a desk, be sure to get up at least once each hour. Take a walk or change positions often.

• Always read in a comfortable position. Rest your arms on your lap, the arms of your chair, a table or a desk while reading.

• Take breaks from any repetitious activity. A housewife suffered severe neck and back pain from doing needlework. Each night while cross-stitching, she held her head slightly to the side and did not support her arms. She remained in the same position for at least five hours each day.

Now, after spending several weeks in a neck brace to reduce the pain, she cross-stitches only for short periods of time.

• Watch your posture. Good posture is important in preventing back strain. Don't slouch or sit in extremely soft chairs or couches. Be sure your back is properly supported whenever you are sitting or lying down. Also, be sure to sit erect with your back not slumped over. When driving or riding in a car, tilt the seat slightly forward. At first this position may feel awkward, but it will give you better support and posture while in the car. When you're working while standing, work at a comfortable level so that you don't have to bend over to reach your work. When lifting objects, try to lift objects using your legs by bending your knees to reach them instead of bending from the back. Avoid sudden movements which twist the body.

• When you're sleeping, a soft mattress is usually the worst thing for back support. If possible, buy a very firm mattress or put a sheet of plywood between your mattress and box springs to give your body extra support.

• Exercise. Regular exercise will help strengthen the back muscles so they will not be strained or aggravated by regular activities. When exercising, try to avoid sudden, jarring movements. Always warm up before starting vigorous exercise and use slow stretching exercises to cool down afterwards. If using aerobic dance for exercise, try low-impact aerobics which keep one foot on the floor at all times, causing less jumping and jarring of the joints. A proper low-impact program will still give a good aerobic workout while lowering the possibility of damaging your back.

• Many cases of back pain occur because people have flat feet or because one leg is shorter than the other. If you have one leg that is shorter than the other, a special shoe can help even out the difference and balance out the forces on your backbone while you're standing. If you have flat feet or poor arches, arch supports can help even out tensions which are transmitted through the leg to the backbone.

• To relieve lower back pain, first lie down and give your back muscles a chance to relax so that the painful spasm can go away. Applications of cold compresses may be helpful. Later on, after the immediate spasm has passed, applications of heat to the area of pain may help to loosen up muscles. Soak in a warm bathtub or apply a heating pad directly to the back. Lie down on a firm surface and relax while applying gentle heat to the area. Try to avoid lying directly on a heating pad. It is best to put the heating pad on top of the body. If you must lie with it underneath, keep the heating pad on the lowest setting and use it for no more than 20 minutes. Soothing ointments which are advertised to help relieve back pain or increase blood flow may also be helpful once the initial spasm has passed. Many doctors also prescribe aspirin to help reduce pain and inflammation during the recovery period.

If you conscientiously follow all the above advice, you can minimize the chance of suffering common backaches if there is not a serious underlying disease which is causing the problem. Developing a lifestyle of taking care of your back may save you a costly visit to the surgeon someday. With back problems, it seems an ounce prevention can be worth a pound of cure.

Exercises That Help The Back

Most back pain occurs because the muscles in the lower back, which help support the spine, are weak from lack of use. Simple exercises which don't strain the back are helpful in building up the strength of these muscles.

• The best gentle back exercise is to lie flat on your back in bed and gradually increase the tension in your abdominal muscles. Next, alternately flatten and then slightly bow your back as you're lying on the bed.

• If you're in fairly good shape, this exercise can help. Stand erect with feet spread apart and slowly bend from the waist until you touch your toes or come close to them. Then, slowly come back to an erect position. With this exercise, the emphasis is on the word "slowly". Sudden movements may cause the very back strain you're trying to guard against. After you've done this exercise for a few days, you can increase the number of repetitions periodically from 5 to 10 to 20 to 30 or more. At this point, your muscles will have gotten stronger so you won't be as likely to strain your back in the future.

• You can also do sit-up exercises to help strengthen the abdominal muscles which help promote good posture. Lie down on the floor with your back flat on the floor and your knees elevated so that your legs slope up at a 45 degree angle. Put your hands on your chest and slowly rise to a sitting position. If this exercise causes strain, just raise your head and shoulders off the ground until this exercise has helped you to get into better shape. At that point, try to do a full sit-up. Again, always sit up with the knees elevated so that the leg forms a 45-degree angle. This elevation of the knees is quite helpful in preventing back strain while doing the exercise.

A Stomach Muscle Exercise That May Hurt Your Back

Depending on how you are exercising to tighten those stomach muscles, you may be "robbing Peter to pay Paul." That is, you may be harming your back to flatten your stomach.

Tony Melles, of the Canadian Back Institute, warns that with many TV gadgets to tighten stomach muscles, people are once again going to be hurting their backs. Since most people who purchase "gut buster" type gadgets on TV are not in good shape, Melles worries that they'll injure their backs while trying to reduce their stomachs.

Straight-legged sit-ups are notoriously bad for your back, and most fitness instructors have switched to bent-knee sit-ups. Doing sit-ups with your knees bent and your feet resting on the floor (not anchored down) is the safest way to help your stomach without hurting your back, Melles explains.

In the end, stronger stomach muscles can give support to your back and help you avoid back pain.

BAD BREATH

Things Your Best Friend May Not
(Know to) Tell You

If you have bad breath, you may be the last to know. How can you tell? Jane Brody, health columnist with the *New York Times*, recommends licking the back of your hand. Wait a couple of minutes and then smell the area, she says. You should be able to determine if your breath is offensive to others. Here are several things to keep in mind if you are plagued by this problem:

• Eating onions or garlic is well-known to cause bad breath, but did you know that what you eat can affect your breath for three days? Not only will food affect your breath as you eat it, but later it is actually absorbed into the bloodstream and the smell of strong odors can still flow from your body.

• Pregnancy, menstruation and ovulation can affect a woman's breath as hormonal changes occur in the body. Doctors suggest that women should become particularly attentive to oral hygiene during pregnancy because the baby is drawing calcium from the mother's body. Without adequate dental care, bad breath and more serious problems can occur.

• **Don't use too much mouthwash.** With saliva and normal eating habits, the body has a built-in mechanism to fight bad breath. Overuse of mouthwashes can harm the body's own natural responses and actually increase the frequency of bad breath. Proper dental care, regular brushing, regular flossing, brushing your tongue, and drinking plenty of water should help keep your mouth and breath sweet.

BIRTH MARKS

Laser Treatment Destroys Birth Marks
without Leaving Scar

A new laser surgery technique has been found effective in at least partially clearing up birth marks while not leaving a scar, according to *Oncology Times*.

Adrianna Scheibner, an Australian dermatologist, shared her technique at the annual meeting of the American Academy of Dermatology. By "reducing the size of the light spot of a low powered laser," birth marks can be treated without damaging the skin, *Oncology Times* reports.

Of three hundred patients with birth marks treated with the new laser, forty-one percent had blemishes almost completely removed, thirty-six percent faded significantly, Scheibner says. Ten percent of the birth marks disappeared completely while thirteen percent faded only slightly.

The size of the light was reduced to almost that of the blood vessels, enabling the laser to pass through the epidermis without breaking the skin. "The lower power tunable laser merely blanched the blood vessels, but did not burn the entire area, so the skin was left intact," Scheibner reports.

Although still in the developmental stage, the laser may eventually be the answer to unwanted birth marks.

BLOOD PRESSURE, HIGH

Tips for Those on
Blood Pressure Medication

Here are some tips for people taking medicine to control high blood pressure:

• Get your blood pressure checked regularly; it takes only a minute or two. If it is above the normal range (140/90), see your doctor.

• Take your prescribed medicine as directed. Keep doing so, because even if you feel better, your high blood pressure is not cured. Regular dosages are necessary to keep it under control.

• Don't change the dose yourself. You might get too much or not enough medicine. Either way it could be harmful. If you take less of your prescription than your doctor prescribes, you may increase the risk of complications such as stroke or heart attack. If you take more of your medication than you're supposed to, you increase the possibility of having side effects from the drug.

• Don't stop taking a drug on your own, even if you feel lightheaded, dizzy, tired, depressed or have trouble sleeping. Your drug can be controlling your blood pressure but may also be giving you these or other side effects. Notify your doctor immediately when bothersome side effects occur. He needs to know how medication is affecting you, in order to treat your condition properly.

• If you have questions about your high pressure or your prescription, don't ask a friend or relative. Their information or advice may be well-intended but wrong for you. Ask your doctor or pharmacist—they are the people qualified to answer.

• Be sure to tell your doctor if you take other medicine regularly. Prescription drugs, vitamins, aspirin and other non-prescription drugs can interact with one another, causing decreased effectiveness or problem side effects.

• Proper diet and exercise often help control high blood pressure. Consult your doctor to see how you can help lower your high blood pressure... maybe to the point where drugs aren't needed!

• People with high blood pressure should avoid overeating when they are on antidepressant drugs. Unusual feelings of hunger and cravings for sweets are experienced by about 50 percent of people taking drugs for depression, according to the journal *Geriatrics* (41:4). The unusual cravings often cause people to eat more than normal and to gain weight. Being overweight is dangerous for everyone, but especially for those with high blood pressure. The pangs of hunger and cravings for sweets seem to be side effects of antidepressant drugs that stop as soon as the drug is discontinued, says the report. If you suspect that your prescription drugs are causing these side effects, discuss them with your doctor. Do *not* stop or change your medicine without your physician's approval.

A Pain Reliever That May Interfere with Your Blood Pressure Medicine

Ibuprofen, an over-the-counter pain reliever, may interfere with prescription drugs controlling blood pressure, according to research by the University of Cincinnati Medical Center (*Annals of Internal Medicine*). Blood pressure levels increased about seven millimeters in just three weeks in patients who took ibuprofen for pain while receiving blood pressure medicine. Increased blood pressure did not occur when aspirin or acetaminophen was used for pain, the study reports.

Ibuprofen is found in many over-the-counter medicines for pain and menstrual camps including Advil®, Haltran®, Ibuprin®, Medipren®, Nuprin®, Pamprin-IB® and Trendar®. Ibuprofen in prescription strengths, used mostly for the pain of arthritis, is available as Ifen®, Motrin®, and Rufen®. The doctors in the study suggest that patients taking any type of blood pressure medicine should refrain from using ibuprofen.

Will Your Children Have High Blood Pressure?

If you suffer, or have suffered, from high blood pressure, be careful with your children's intake of salt, according to research published in the journal *Pediatrics*.

Craving salt is an acquired taste. Do not salt your children's food. Limit the amount of salt you use in food preparation. Limit the children's intake of highly salted foods like canned soups, potato chips, pickles and cured meats. If children do not grow up with salt, they will not crave it, and you will lower their risk of getting high blood pressure in the future.

High Blood Pressure? One of Four Are Wrongly Diagnosed

Have you been diagnosed as having high blood

pressure? You may want to get another reading.

Researchers in Canada found that "one of every four people who appeared to have high blood pressure actually did not," according to *Prevention* magazine.

Dr. Nicholas Birkett, the study's chief researcher, speculates that those people experienced "white-coat apprehension" — nervousness at being in the presence of a doctor or nurse. This caused their blood pressure to be unusually high during the doctor's office reading.

When blood pressure was taken twice more on two separate occasions, the people were found to have normal blood pressure.

Birkett's findings have been confirmed by investigators at Cornell University Medical Center. They compared blood pressure measurements obtained by doctors with readings taken by an automatic arm recorder worn during the day. For both hypertension patients and those with normal blood pressure "the highest blood pressure recorded was the one taken by the physician," according to *Harvard Medical School Health Letter*.

For an accurate diagnosis of mild high blood pressur Dr. Birkett recommends taking three or four separate readings over as long as six months.

Lower Blood Pressure
by the Way You Talk?

High blood pressure is related to diverse factors like age, weight, stress, smoking, talking. Talking?

That's right. Research suggests your blood pressure can shoot up simply by "shooting the breeze."

James J. Lynch, Ph.D., a psychology professor at the University of Maryland School of Medicine, maintains that the act of speaking, regardless of what's being said, can raise blood pressure high enough "it creates the appearance of hypertension" (*Medical Tribune*).

Based on research over the last eight years, Lynch is convinced that communication raises blood pressure. He believes patients with hypertension can be taught to curb the malady by speaking differently.

Talking itself is certainly not unhealthy, Lynch says. His research shows, however, that certain mechanical factors such as how you breathe influences high blood pressure. Lynch notes that hypertensives often "talk breathlessly." By teaching them to "slow down the rate of speech, speaking with a listener in mind," he says, hypertensives can be guided by doctors toward lower blood pressure.

Lynch admits more research is necessary to determine what really happens to the cardiovascular system during speech. Yet the connection between increased blood pressure and speech is more than a theory, he claims, it's a law.

In other words, says Lynch, "dialogue is truly heartfelt."

Float Away High Blood Pressure

A man suffering from hypertension and high blood pressure enters what looks like a Porsche without wheels. Actually it is a tank with no windows, filled with densely salted water. When the hatch is closed he lies back and floats effortlessly in the buoyant water, which is heated to body temperature. The tank is pitch dark and soundproof, and he has the feeling of being suspended in time and space. Tensions gently ebb away.

Flotation centers, whether they use a Porsche-like water tank or just an overgrown bathtub in a dark, soundproof room, are becoming the rage, according to *Psychology Today* . An hour session runs from $20 to $30.

Doctors call the treatment Restricted

Environmental Stimulation Therapy, or REST. Studies have shown it not only relaxes people with hypertension, but reduces their blood pressure as well.

Neuroendocrinologist John W. Turner, Jr., and clinical psychologist Thomas H. Fine at the Medical College of Ohio found that after 20 flotation sessions a patient's blood pressure was reduced. Hormones related to stress also decreased in most cases, and heart and respiration rates dropped.

Psychology Today cites a study of 20 borderline hypertensives at the State University at Stoney Brook. The study found blood pressure decreased after floating once or twice a week for five weeks.

REST has also been known to reduce pain in rheumatoid arthritis sufferers. Some research suggests it can even enhance learning ability.

How does it work? No one knows for sure, but Peter Suedfeld of the University of British Columbia has an idea about why it is effective in reducing blood pressure. Suedfeld says it has to do with focus.

By necessity we pay more attention to external information than internal. During REST however, there is no external material to deal with. Instead attention is "focused on the internally generated material," Suedfeld says.

Turner adds that when the normal bombardment of external stimuli we constantly face is removed, the body adjusts itself to a new, optimal blood pressure 'set point.'

The bottom line is: Life today is demanding and offers constant external stimulation; we need a break or, as Suedfeld puts it, a "going away." Suedfeld feels the more demanding a society, the greater the need for a period of "going away-ness." REST is just what the doctor orders.

High Blood Pressure?
Listen to This!

Talking too much may irritate your friends, but did you know it could also be hazardous to your health? One research study shows that listening, rather than talking, lowers blood pressure. Most people experience a rise in blood pressure when they speak, followed by a rapid drop when they listen, reports *Arteries Cleaned Out Naturally* .

The study indicates that the louder and faster a person talks, the higher the blood pressure. (See the article "Lower Blood Pressure by the Way You Talk?) Learning to listen may reduce stress and the load on the heart.

So the next time you visit your friends, listen to what they have to say. It will not only help them, it will also do your own heart good.

BLOOD PRESSURE, LOW

Be Careful About
That Shower!

Before you shower after exercising, cool down, warns Dr. John Cantwell in the *American Medical Journal* (252:429). Cantwell, the team doctor for the Atlanta Braves baseball club, says that showering too soon after exercising can cause spasms in your arteries or a sharp decrease in blood pressure.

Exercise causes a fall in blood pressure because the blood tends to collect in the legs after exercising, he explains. If you take a hot or warm shower while in this condition, the hot water can dilate the blood vessels.

On the other hand, a cold shower can raise blood pressure and place a sudden strain on the heart. This could cause some arteries to go into spasms, explains the doctor. To avoid any bad effects, Dr. Cantwell says that after exercising you should completely cool down before heading for the showers.

BONE HEALING

A Forthcoming Source
of Healing

Electromedicine is making important strides in improving healing, says Dr. Andrew L Bassett, professor of orthopedic surgery at Columbia University. Bassett says that electromagnetic pulses, sent from a small battery pack worn outside your clothing, can help heal broken bones, hip disintegration, tendonitis and may even be useful against osteoporosis.

Pulsed electromagnetic fields (PEMF) are now being used to heal broken bones that have not improved during normal treatment, he explained. The PEMF units are usually worn on a belt and a wire from the battery pack is attached directly to the injured area. Bassett hopes that nightly PEMF treatments could be used in the future to help heal bones while people are sleeping, therefore preventing or reducing osteoporosis.

BREATHING PROBLEMS

Spicy Foods Help Aging Lungs

A Mexican dinner or a take-out order of spicy Chinese food is just what this doctor orders for aging lungs.

As we get older, respiration becomes more difficult. That's because the total surface area of lung tissue is reduced and the muscles that move the chest wall during breathing become weaker, according to *Prevention* magazine. Even minor respiratory ailments can be dangerous for an older person.

While getting enough nutrients such as vitamins A, C and E, can help prevent respiratory problems that threaten the elderly, the kind of food you eat is just as important.

Lung specialist Irwin Ziment, M.D., of the Los Angeles County-Olive View Medical Center in California, has found that eating spicy foods seems to be a good way to help patients clear lung congestion, *Prevention* reports.

"Probably everyone's experienced the phenomenon when they eat spicy meals at a Szechwan Chinese restaurant, or an Indian or Mexican restaurant," Ziment says. "They get watery eyes, runny nose or even sneezing. If we paid close attention, we'd notice that it's easier to cough up mucus in those situations."

People with respiratory problems often have a buildup of mucus in the lungs.

"Spicy foods stimulate the stomach and cause a reflex action in the lungs, which results in the excretion of fluids," Ziment says.

CANCER

You May Be Able to Beat It After All!

Beating cancer may be as simple as a blood test. Dr. Eric Fossel of Harvard University has produced a new blood test that can spot cancer as small as one-eighth of an inch. The blood test will help doctors save thousands of lives because it identifies cancer early (when most treatable) no matter where it is located in the body.

Fossel estimates that the cost for each test will be inexpensive, perhaps $20.00. However, the machine used to read the test, a nuclear magnetic resonace (NMR) spectrometer, is worth about $400,000. Over three thousand people have had the blood test with a 95 percent rate of accuracy, Fossel explains. The blood test may be available to doctors around the country within a few years.

Another sign of hope is that a vaccine to prevent melanoma skin cancer may not be far away. Dr. Jean Claude Bystryn at the Kaplan Cancer Center of New York University Medical Center has created a vaccine that increases immunity in animals. Dr. Bystryn says the study took seven years, and it will be several more years before it could be ready for use in people.

Although the safety has been established, more tests will be needed to determine its effectiveness in preventing life-threatening melanoma or in preventing the progression of the disease.

This Nutrient Helps Prevent Lung Cancer

For generations children have been encouraged, cajoled and forced by their parents to eat carrots because of the supposed benefits to the eyes. Research now suggests that the vitamin A found in carrots does a lot more than enhance eyesight: it may help prevent lung cancer.

A study at the State University of New York at Buffalo compared the diets of 900 healthy people with that of 450 lung cancer patients. Researchers found that those with lung cancer ingested much less beta-carotene than the healthy people, according to *Prevention* magazine.

Beta-carotene, found in large quantities in carrots, is converted by the body to vitamin A. Vitamin A helps maintain the epithelial tissue that lines part of the lungs. It is thought either beta-carotene directly "protects the lungs from cancer," *Prevention* says, or that "vitamin A squelches free radicals." (Free radicals are the compounds in the body which are thought to trigger cancer).

The difference between the beta-carotene intake of those with high and low risks of cancer "amounted to about 6,750 international units (IU), the amount provided by a single carrot," *Prevention* reports.

New Test Warns of Lung Cancer
Before It's Too Late

"By the time lung cancer shows up on an x-ray, it's usually too late," *Prevention* magazine says. The article adds that a new sputum test called Novacyte can reveal precancerous changes in the lungs before cancer takes hold.

"The test may help millions of smokers by showing lung-cell changes that could lead to or indicate cancer far earlier than x-rays can," the article says.

The test is available by prescription. After taking it home and administering the test yourself, you mail the sputum specimen to the manufacturer, Xsirius Medical Inc. They will analyze it and send the results to your doctor. If you don't have a doctor, they will connect you with one as long as you are a smoker, over 40 and have a chronic cough.

Of course, if the test reveals lung cancer is imminent, the choice is simple: quit smoking or contract the disease. The test won't make that decision any easier, but it gives you fair warning before it's too late.

The peace of mind the test provides can make it worth the $90 it costs.

Cancer Prevention Tips

• Avoid drinking or cooking with chlorinated water.

• Avoid using talcum powder in the genital areas.

• Avoid coffee: regular or decaffeinated.

• Avoid contact with asbestos.

• Avoid excessive exposure to the sun.

• Avoid fried foods.

• Avoid processed foods containing additives which have been found to contribute to the development of cancer.

• Avoid barrier forms of contraception.

• Eat foods rich in vitamin D, calcium, molybdenum and selenium, such as fish, whole grain foods, wheat germ and beans.

• Include lysine in your diet.

• Eat crunchy yellow and dark green leafy vegetables.

• Reduce the amount of sodium in your diet

and increase the amount of potassium.
- Eat foods containing high dietary fiber.
- Avoid cigarettes.
- Avoid excessive use of alcohol.

Can Repressed Emotions Increase Your Chances of Dying of Cancer?

After enduring a painful divorce behind a cheerful mask, a Connecticut school teacher developed breast and, later, bone cancer. Her doctor informed her family she would soon die.

Today "more assertive and expressive," she has apparently weathered the cancer storm, according to *Psychology Today*.

"I feel the cancer is related to the repression of my feelings and to chronic stress," she says.

For 25 years researchers have tried to connect emotions, stress or personality traits to a person's chances of developing or surviving cancer. Emotions are not easily defined, and researchers' findings have been as varied as their methods. A recent study, however, suggests a strong link between repressed emotions and the ability of a person to fight cancer.

Two psychologists at Johns Hopkins University School of Medicine studied the personality traits and health records of students between 1948 and

71

1964, *Psychology Today* reports. The men were divided into five groups based on personality traits.

The most cancer-free group was the "Acting Out/Emotional cluster"—people who expressed their emotions, however negative. Even a group with a positive outlook on life, who nevertheless held anxiety inside, was more likely to develop cancer than the Acting Out/Emotional cluster.

The group designated the "Loner Cluster" had the highest incidence of cancer. These people met life with an unemotional stoicism and often felt lonely.

"The trait common to most of the clusters with higher cancer rates is a tendency to hide real feelings, particularly negative ones," *Psychology Today* concludes.

The Johns Hopkins study confirmed results of a 1985 study of breast cancer patients at King's College Hospital in Ontario, Canada. Patients who either fought the disease or denied the diagnosis were more likely to survive five to ten years than those who stoically accepted their disease or felt hopeless and helpless.

New Haven, Connecticut, surgeon Bernie Siegal is one of the few doctors outspoken in his belief that repressed emotions and feelings of helplessness contribute to a higher risk of cancer and shortened life. He is critical of the way doctors give patients a grim prognosis that often sounds like a death sentence at what is most likely the most devastating point of their lives.

"Instead of turning fighters into victims, we should be turning victims into fighters," Siegal says.

University of Pennsylvania psychologist Barrie Cassileth, however, offers another side. In a 1985 study of patients in advanced or intermediate stages of cancer, she found no link between attitudes, length of survival, or remission. Cassileth also believes it is dangerous to encourage denial of the prognosis as it may encourage patients to avoid medical treatment for unproven, potentially harmful therapies.

"The bottom line is that cancer is an overwhelming biological event in which psychological or social factors play a minor role," says Cassileth. She admits though, that medical treatments often don't work.

Until more research is done, a dose of Cassileth's realism should probably be taken by cancer patients along with a liberal portion of Siegal's advice to express what they feel about the disease and never give in to it.

Train Your Immune System
To Fight Cancer?

Can you actually train your immune system to fight cancer? It may be possible, say researchers at the University of Alabama.

They reached their conclusions after using conditioning procedures on mice much as Pavlov used with a dog. (It was Pavlov who discovered a dog would salivate at the sound of a bell after being conditioned to associate the sound with food.)

According to *Prevention* magazine the Alabama researchers trained mice to produce interferon (which activates natural killer cells, our body': first line of defense against cancer) after exposing them to the smell of camphor. The researchers injected the mice with an interferon-stimulating chemical, then exposed them to the camphor odor for four hours every three days for 27 days. After the 27 days, some mice were exposed to the camphor smell without receiving an injection. They still produced "three times more interferon...and killer cell activity than mice that were not exposed," the article reports.

Does this mean our immune systems can be conditioned to respond to a pleasant smell or maybe a particular melody? The Alabama researchers say that is their "ultimate hope."

The research team organizer says, "we know from studies regarding stress, grief and happiness, that the immune system is linked to the central nervous system. Now we are beginning to see how we can influence that interaction."

Based on their experiment with mice, the researchers hope the immune system of a cancer patient can eventually be trained to copy the effect of immune-stimulating drugs.

Warning: This Drink May Cause Cancer

A potent carcinogen called urethane is present in hundreds of alcoholic beverages, the *Nutrition Action Health Letter* says. Worse, no one seems to know how to remove it from the beverages.

According to government tests, the most highly contaminated are bourbon whiskey and fruit brandies. "But many dessert wines, table wines and liqueurs are also tainted," the *Letter* adds. The Food and Drug Administration has yet to publicize the names of brands containing urethane.

The Center for Science in the Public Interest (CSPI), however, has put out a booklet entitled "Tainted Booze" which lists the levels of contamination in over 1,100 brand name products.

It also answers questions about urethane. The booklet's author, Charles Mitchell, says that although the whiskey and wine industries have agreed to lower levels of urethane in their future products, they are still too high.

"There is no evidence that any safe level of urethane can be ingested without increasing the risk of cancer," he adds.

So far the whiskey and wine industries' agreement to set limits on the amounts of urethane they put in their products is voluntary; there is no way of assuring they stick to their guns. Also, the agreements do not protect consumers from urethane-contaminated booze now being sold, the *Nutrition Action Health Letter* points out.

Coffee and Cigarettes:
A Deadly Combination

"Cancer of the pancreas is the fourth leading cause of cancer death in the U.S.," reports *The Western Journal of Medicine*.

Coffee has often been cited as a possible cause of pancreatic cancer. A recent study by five doctors in southern California did find a link between coffee intake and cancer of the pancreas, the *Journal* says. But the study showed that coffee drinkers who smoked faced the greatest risk.

Previous studies have focused on either cigarettes or coffee as risk factors. This controlled study, conducted in a county near San Diego, divided the coffee drinking participants into smokers and non-smokers.

Results showed that while the risk of pancreatic cancer is fairly low in those who drink less than four cups of coffee a day, those who both smoke cigarettes and drink coffee stand a much greater chance of getting pancreatic cancer.

Interestingly, the results were basically the same regardless of whether a person drank regular or decaffeinated coffee.

"This study is the first to show an effect of drinking coffee on the risk of pancreatic cancer that is almost completely limited to cigarette smokers," the *Journal* concludes.

Skin Cancer from
Driving Your Car?

It is common knowlege that exposure to too much sun can cause skin cancer. Doctors consider sunscreen essential for prolonged stays at the beach or tennis court. But did you ever think of applying sunscreen before a ride in the car?

A study of 766 people with solar keratoses

(skin growths often a sign of imminent skin cancer) at Monash University in Australia, seemed to confirm a pattern doctors have long observed linking skin cancer to automobile driving, *Prevention* magazine reports.

Doctors noticed keratoses and skin cancer to be more frequent on the left side of people in the United States and on the right side of people in Australia and Great Britain (where the steering wheel is on the right). They have attributed this to the greater amount of sunlight people are exposed to when they drive with the window open.

The Australian study revealed that men had many more keratoses on their right forearms and hands than on their left, because until recently most drivers in Australia were men. Keratoses afflicted women primarily on the left side of the neck and head, since women passengers often sit lower in the seat than men, exposing more of their heads and necks to the sun.

The moral, doctors say, is: Use sunscreen before long or frequent rides in the car with the window open.

Warning to Industrial Workers: This Chemical Can Cause Cancer

Seven aircraft repairmen and three leather

tanners were recently diagnosed as having testicular cancer. The ten workers had one thing in common: exposure to dimethylformamide (DMF).

At least 100,000 workers in the United States are exposed to the chemical DMF. This chemical is used as a solvent in leather dyes and pesticides as well as in the production of paint, artificial fibers and drugs.

The *Harvard Medical School Health Letter* reports that DMF has caused "testicular abnormalities and possibly cancer in laboratory animals." Although it has not yet been proven to cause cancer in humans, doctors consider it a significant risk factor.

The *Health Letter* advises workers to minimize exposure to DMF as well as to perform monthly self-examinations. And for good reason: Testicular cancer is the most common form of cancer among young adult men in the United States.

Cancer from Your Wood-burning Stove?

The energy crisis of the 1970's helped make wood-burning stoves the most popular fad since the hula-hoop. Still gracing many American family rooms, they speak of simpler times, before cancer was a known threat.

Now even the wood-burning stove is being implicated as a source of carcinogens, according to *Health and Enviroment Digest* .

The state of Maine has determined that wood smoke is a "priority public health concern," according to the *Digest*. It bases its assessment on a study of the risks of wood smoke drafted by the state's Bureau of Health.

The investigators noted that many of wood smoke's chemical components are known carcinogens. "There is reason to be concerned about long-term, low-level exposure to wood smoke," the researchers concluded.

Maine's Bureau of Public Health is continuing to study the risks of exposure to smoke from wood-burning stoves and will begin assessing the "impacts of complex mixtures in wood smoke," the article concludes.

CARPAL TUNNEL SYNDROME

Help for Hurting Hands

The twist of the wrist required in the simplest of tasks such as opening a door can cause searing pain for a Carpal Tunnel Syndrome (CTS) sufferer.

"An estimated one in ten Americans will develop CTS," *Prevention* magazine says. It is a condition which can lead to complete loss of mobility in the hand.

"Carpal Tunnel Syndrome occurs when the tendons, bones or ligaments in the wrist press against the median nerve, short-circuiting it," the article says. The median nerve is the path that nerve impulses take on their trip from the spinal cord through the arm and wrist and into the fingers. Most of the sensation in the hand as well as the muscle power of the thumb is supplied by the median nerve.

Usually the bones and ligaments in the wrist form a "protective sheath or 'tunnel' around the nerve and tendons," *Prevention* says. When someone has CTS, "it's as if you laid a two-by-four down" on top of the tunnel, thereby hampering the flow of nerve impulses, neurologist Colin Hall, M.D., explains.

The first signs of Carpal Tunnel Syndrome are numbness, pain, weakness and a "pins and needles" sensation in the thumb and fingers. Often these symptoms are more noticeable at night.

The cause of Carpal Tunnel Syndrome is unknown, although a clue can be found in the types of jobs or tasks many sufferers have. Those people with jobs requiring repetitious manual motions, such as meat cutters, cashiers and assembly line workers face the highest risk. Homemakers who sew, knit or wring wet laundry also have a better-than-average chance of getting it.

Women are twice as susceptible to CTS as men, perhaps because their wrists, and therefore their carpal "tunnels," are narrower than men's. Pregnant women in particular are more likely to suffer from CTS. Diabetes, arthritis and menopause are also risk factors.

For most people, CTS is painful and annoying but not incapacitating. Surgery, therefore, should be turned to only if the following therapies have failed:

• First, learn to use your hands in ways that don't put pressure on the median nerve, *Prevention* counsels. Just as what you do contributes to CTS, how you do it can keep the problem in check. By counseling factory workers

82

on how to reduce the risk of injuring their wrists, Glenda Key has "reduced the incidence of CTS by as much as 94 percent," *Prevention* reports. Imparting what she calls "worker's wisdom" to housewives as well as factory workers, Key has taught the proper methods for doing everything from brushing hair to putting plates in a cupboard.

"Our focus is on teaching people how to use their hands in a safer, easier, more comfortable way," Key says.

• Another option is a forearm splint. A splint enforces hand rest, allowing it to heal. Some people have experienced relief from pain only 24 hours after donning the splint. Splints are available in medical supply stores or they can be custom-fitted by physical or occupational therapists, according to *The Western Journal of Medicine*. The custom-fitted splints are lighter and less clumsy than the store-bought variety.

• A third option involves vitamin B6 supplements. The vitamin is "widely publicized as a treatment for CTS," *Prevention* says, but the medical community is still skeptical about its supposed benefits.

John M. Ellis, M.D., of Mount Pleasant, Texas, believes B6 deficiency brings on CTS symptoms. He claims to have cured CTS sufferers with B6 doses one hundred times the Recommended

Dietary Allowance. No other research on this subject, however, has yet been conducted, and there have been reports linking loss of feeling in the limbs and nerve damage to high intakes of vitamin B6.

Surgery should only be considered if the above treatment options have failed or if there is a risk of permanent damage to nerves and muscles of the hand.

CATARACTS

Natural Ways to Prevent Cataracts

Cataracts occur when the lens of the eye becomes cloudy, often with advancing age. It may start when an enzyme system, which helps keep the lens of the eye clear, performs less efficiently with age. Factors contributing to the development of cataracts are:

• Exposure to ultraviolet light. Wearing sunglasses in bright sunlight or avoiding bright sunlight may be helpful in preventing cataracts.

• Riboflavin (vitamin B2) deficiency may be one cause of cataracts. There are reports of cataracts diminishing after supplements of riboflavin were taken, but these claims are unconfirmed at this time. On the other hand, taking large doses of the vitamin niacin (vitamin B3) or other B vitamins may increase the chances of getting cataracts.

Additional vitamin C has been found to lower the risk of cataracts, according to a study at Tufts University by Allan Taylor, M.D. Vitamin C seems to stop cataracts by blocking the proteins that form cataracts on the lens of the eye. High amounts of vitamin C are naturally found in uncooked rose hips, acerola cherries, citrus fruits, green peppers, parsley, broccoli, brussels sprouts, cabbage and potatoes.

A recent study has also shown that people who regularly take acetaminophen or aspirin have one-half the rate of cataracts as people who don't take them.

CHOLESTEROL

Tips For Reducing Cholesterol

High levels of cholesterol may lead to arteriosclerosis, or hardening of the arteries, which in turn may impede blood flow to the heart and perhaps cause a heart attack. According to the National Institute of Health (NIH), every one percent reduction in total cholesterol leads to a two percent reduction in the risk of developing coronary heart disease. The NIH recommends that all adults bring their total cholesterol levels down below 200 mg/dl.

Here are some facts to consider about cholesterol reduction:

• Reducing cholesterol with the drug gemfibrozil (brand name Lopid®) has been proven to reduce the incidence of heart disease, according the five-year Helsinki Heart Study published in *The New England Journal of Medicine* (317:20, 1237). Before now, cholesterol-reducing drugs were only "thought" to help fight heart-disease but conclusive studies had not been completed. The researchers found the decrease in heart disease after the first year of treatment with 600 mg. of gemfibrozil twice daily. However, in the five years there was no difference in the overall death rate or cancer rate when compared to a control group who didn't receive the drug.

• A common, over-the-counter laxative has been proven to reduce cholesterol. Metamucil® reduced total cholesterol levels by 15 percent in just eight weeks, according to a study by James Anderson, M.D., at the University of Kentucky College of Medicine (reported in the *Archives of Internal Medicine*). Participants took 3.4 grams of Metamucil® three times a day and significantly lowered their cholesterol. Metamucil®, technically known as psyllium hydrophillic mecilloid, is made from the husks of blond psyllium seeds. Dr. Anderson decided to study psyllium because it is a water-soluble fiber similar to guar gum, oat gum and pectin. "These preliminary results indicate that Metamucil® may help the millions of people whose cholesterol levels put them at risk for coronary heart disease," Dr. Anderson says. Other products that contain psyllium as the active ingredient are Alramucil®, Effersyllium®, Fiberall®, Hydrocil®, Modane Versabran®, Naturacil®, Perdium®, Prompt® and Syllact®.

• Eat fish just three times a week and lower your risk of heart and artery problems, according to Dragoslava Vesselinovitch, D.V.M., from the

University of Chicago School of Medicine. Even if you have a high fat diet, eating fish will help reduce your cholesterol levels, Vesselinovitch says. But eating fish more often will not increase the benefits. Three times a week seems to be the optimum amount.

• Are you eating the right kind of fiber? Americans are increasing the amount of fiber in their diets but only certain types of dietary fiber help to lower cholesterol. Water-soluble fibers, like pectin and guar gum, are the only type of fiber that helps reduce cholesterol, Dr. Ann L. Gerhardt of the University of California-Davis Medical Center explains. Wheat bran contains a non-soluble form of fiber so it doesn't help in the cholesterol battle. Pectin is found in many fruits, like pears and apples. Guar gum is contained in oat bran, oatmeal, rolled oats, and many beans. Increase your consumption of kidney beans, pinto beans, garbanzo beans, chickpeas, navy beans, lentils, all fruits and vegetables and oat bran. Wheat bran and foods containing non-soluble fiber are still important to a well-balanced diet but you should know that they aren't involved in decreasing cholesterol.

• Education may help prevent or reduce heart problems. A five-year study of school children showed improved health and awareness in those who were taught the importance of diet, physical activity and not smoking, the *New England Journal of Medicine* (318:17, 1093) says. Since the "natural history of coronary heart disease begins in youth," the researchers hope the widespread education could help reduce the cholesterol levels in children and provide the basis for a healthy generation.

Odorless Garlic:
Lower Blood Fat
without Losing Friends

Eating large amounts of garlic is recognized by doctors as effective in helping the body lose harmful blood fats. Unfortunately, eating that much garlic may cause you to lose most of your friends as well.

Now there's a solution. Kyolic, a product from Japan advertised as "odor-modified, color aged," apparently lowers blood fats without the odoriferous side effects, according to *Prevention* magazine.

A study at Loma Linda University in California measured the effects of the new garlic on blood fat levels o f people with moderately high blood cholesterol levels. The participants in the study were given four capsules, one gram each, of the liquid garlic extract each day.

The "lipid levels" of most patients dropped an average of 44 points after six months, *Prevention* reports. The study's main researcher, Benjamen Lau, says that cholesterol, triglycerides, and low and very low-density lipoproteins (LDL's) all dropped, while beneficial high-density lipoproteins (HDL's) rose. Apparently garlic inhibits the liver's production of harmful blood fats, he adds.

The key to garlic's benefits lies in its most active anti-clotting ingredient, ajoene, according to Eric Block, Ph.D., of the State University of New York at Albany. Block says the ingredient apparently changes "the surface membranes of platelet cells so they're less likely to stick together."

Lau warns that garlic will not prevent heart disease if your diet still includes a lot of saturated fats. Taken with a low-fat diet, however, garlic appears to be helpful in clearing out arteries. And thanks to kyolic, you need no longer fear clearing out a room of people after taking it.

Peanut Butter and Jelly Sandwich Raises Cholesterol Levels?

Other than Mom's apple pie, perhaps no

American staple is as loved and cherished as the peanut butter and jelly sandwich. This luncheon standby couldn't possibly be harmful, could it?

Unfortunately there is evidence that peanut oil, which accounts for 80 percent of peanut butter's calories, might lead to atherosclerosis, the blocking of arteries with cholesterol plaque, the *Nutrition Action Health Letter* reports. Studies so far have been limited to animals, however.

These studies will come as a surprise to some who consider peanut oil harmless because it is mostly unsaturated and therefore should not raise blood cholesterol levels.

Yet back in the 1970's, Robert Wissler of the University of Chicago observed that diets high in peanut oil clogged the arteries of Rhesus monkeys more than did butterfat.

Wissler's experiments have been questioned because he included so much cholesterol in the monkeys' diets. Researchers have claimed the clogged arteries of the monkeys was due primarily to the cholesterol, not the peanut oil.

Wissler counters that high amounts of cholesterol were needed to simulate the amount people ingest over many years, since atherosclerosis generally requires one-third to one-half of a life span to develop in humans. This is the equivalent of five to ten years in primates.

Wissler also points out that the same amount of cholesterol was used with the other fats tested (butter fat and corn oil) as with the peanut oil. Peanut oil did more damage than the other fats.

On the other hand the *Nutrition Action Health Letter* notes that peanut oil clearly lowers the "bad" LDL cholesterol and cites the low incidence of heart disease among the Chinese (peanut oil is a staple in China). But since their diet includes so little cholesterol and fats of all types, damage caused by peanut oil may be undetectable.

The *Nutrition Action Health Letter* recommends caution. It is better not to use peanut oil as a staple for cooking until more tests are done. But thankfully the evidence does not yet suggest resorting to "tofu and jelly sandwiches."

The Best Mealtime
Cholesterol Preventative

Garbanzos, kidney beans and cowpeas are not celebrity foods. But they just might be your best mealtime friends nutrition-wise.

Legumes (or beans) are good sources of iron, magnesium, zinc, protein and several B vitamins, according to the Tufts University *Diet and*

Nutrition Letter. In these respects, they are similar to meat and poultry.

Unlike meat, however, "they are practically devoid of fat, free of cholesterol," the *Letter* says. In addition, beans are highest of all foods in soluble fiber, which is now believed to lower blood cholesterol levels and thereby reduce the risk for developing heart disease.

In light of their impressive contributions, beans should be consumed for nutritional reasons alone. Yet beans are also inexpensive and easy to serve in a variety of ways.

"Legumes combine just as well with vegetables and grains as meats do," the *Letter* says. Also they store easily, and "at a fraction of the price of meat, they are among the best high-protein food bargains you can buy."

Walk Away From
Cholesterol Problems

"You don't have to be a marathoner to be healthy," says Timothy Cook, Ph.D. Leading a team of researchers at the University of Pittsburgh, Cook discovered that the level of the beneficial HDL cholesterol, which reduces the risk of heart disease, was higher in men who exercised regularly, albeit moderately, than in men who lived more sedentary lives, according to *Prevention* magazine.

A comparison was made between the HDL levels of a group of inactive men and those of a group of men who exercised moderately on a regular basis. The latter was a group of 35 mailmen who walked an average of five miles a day in the space of four to five hours.

HDL levels were higher in the mailmen. Their HDL2 cholesterol level, "a specific and beneficial type of HDL," *Prevention* says, was also much greater.

These findings are significant in light of prevalent ideas that hard-core aerobic exercise is necessary for proper fitness.

Cook concludes that "HDL is more affected by chronic activity than by physiological (aerobic) fitness." While not down-playing the importance of aerobic fitness in lowering risk of disease, Cook believes you can also "reduce your risk by being moderately active each day; doing things such as walking."

CIRCULATION

Help for Poor Circulation

Vitamin E has an anticoagulant effect that may help prevent certain circulation problems. It has been used to treat people with intermittent claudication, those with poor circulation in the legs, and people who have a tendency to have leg cramps and form blood clots in the legs.

Niacin is a vasodilator (blood-vessel enlarger). It may improve circulation in the elderly and help keep arms and legs from falling asleep. The effectiveness of this use is unknown, and it may vary.

In diabetics, chromium supplements may aid in treating poor circulation.

Any vitamin or mineral supplements beyond the recommended daily dietary allowance (RDA) may cause harmful side effects and should only be taken with a physician's approval.

COLITIS

Dietary Help for
Colitis Sufferers

The term colitis refers to a number of diseases, all characterized by inflammation of the colon— the lower and biggest part of the large intestine. The inflamation can cause gas, stomach cramps and bloody stools. In severe cases a person may be unable to pass waste from the body.

According to the Tufts University *Diet and Nutrition Letter*, the exact causes of colitis are not known. Treatments therefore sometimes differ. Many doctors, however, agree that dietary treatments can be extremely helpful.

The Tufts University letter recommends a low-fiber diet for colitis sufferers. Raw fruits and vegetables, bran and whole grains should be cut back sharply if not entirely. Such measures will lessen irritation of the colon. (It is hoped they will decrease the frequency of bathroom visits as well.) Nutritional supplements may also be needed, the letter adds; when suffering from colitis a person may have little appetite and therefore may not be consuming adequate nutrients through food.

The Saturday Evening Post recommends a dairy product-free diet for colitis sufferers. Many colitis victims suffer from a reaction to lactose in dairy products which they don't digest properly.

CONSTIPATION

Exercise and Slower Lifestyle
Eliminate More Than Stress

Constipation is caused by many things. One cause not commonly recognized is irritable bowel syndrome, a digestive tract disorder often confused with colitis. Unlike colitis, irritable bowel syndrome is apparently not a result of a physical disorder, according to the Tufts University *Diet and Nutrition Letter*. Rather it is believed to be brought on by emotional stress.

Doctors often call irritable bowel syndrome "spastic colon" because of the painful colon contractions that characterize it, the *Letter* reports. These contractions result in "alternating constipation and diarrhea, sometimes accompanied by nausea, heartburn, and fatigue."

Irritable bowel syndrome usually affects "type A" personalities, particularly those under a lot of stress who eat hurriedly and don't get enough sleep.

High fiber diets are recommended to help the formation of softer stools that are easy to pass (except during diarrhea phases). Coffee, alchohol, spices and gassy foods like beans may make symptoms worse and therefore should be avoided.

Regular exercise to keep the colon muscles in tone is also recommended.

Perhaps most important, however, is a change in lifestyle to reduce stress. As the *Letter* says, quite often "when the stress goes away, the symptoms go away."

DENTAL PROBLEMS

Chewing This Vitamin
Can Destroy Your Teeth

Do you need additional vitamin C? Certainly there are many health benefits from it.

However, dentists are now recommending that if you take a vitamin C supplement, you should take the kind that can be swallowed whole, rather than using chewable tablets. They report that since vitamin C is an acid (ascorbic acid) it can destroy tooth enamel when exposed to the teeth for long periods of time (*Journal of the American Medical Association* 107:253).

Chew Away Cavities

While consuming candy and chewing gum will usually earn you a quick trip to the dentist, there's one "treat" that might keep the dentist away.

The University of Michigan Dental School conducted a study to determine the cavity-fighting ability of chewing gum sweetened with xylitol, *Prevention* magazine reports. Xylitol is a "natural sugar obtained from fruits, vegetables and birch bark."

Cavity-prone children who chewed the gum three times a day had up to 80 percent fewer new cavities than a similar group of children who did not chew the gum, *Prevention* reports.

Kauko Makinen, Ph.D., who conducted the study, says that xylitol was actually superior to fluoride in preventing new cavities. He explains that the sweetener "interferes with the growth of the microorganisms that form plaque," loosens plaque and allows easier removal by brushing.

"I think xylitol gum and flouride treatment could be a very effective combination in preventing cavities," Makinen concludes.

However, one side effect of chewing xylitol gum is a coated tongue, according to an earlier study.

Heart Damage after Dental Visits

Considering the discomfort a thorough teeth-cleaning at the dentist's office can cause, it may come as no surprise that infections sometimes occur. But in the lining of the heart?

Dental procedures and infection of the gums and teeth are the most frequent known cause of infection of the heart lining, according to *Heartline* newsletter.

Germs often enter the bloodstream following dental procedures. A person with an abnormal heart valve, who is therefore easily subject to an infection of the heart lining, can be plagued by any wayward germ entering the blood stream. After a dental visit a germ might get into the blood stream and "settle on a damaged heart valve, set up housekeeping, and cause serious infection," *Heartline* says.

The newsletter recommends that those with valvular heart disease practice "the best oral hygiene possible." Infection could result from simple neglect, causing bloodstream infection even before going to the dentist.

For those with an abnormal heart valve, the American Heart Association suggests taking an antibiotic before any dental procedure which may cause gum bleeding, including cleaning. Patients who have had heart valve infections previously or have artificial heart valves will require two antibiotic injections one hour before the dental procedure.

A different antibiotic is available for those allergic to penicillin. This must be injected directly into the vein. Blood thinning pills must be discontinued for several days before the dental procedure to prevent bleeding into muscle injection sites.

Heartline adds that those with no previous heart infections or no artificial heart valves can take antibiotic pills in lieu of injections.

Smile, No More Cavities or Costly Dental Bills

Has your dentist told you? Tooth decay can be prevented by a procedure as easy and painless as a manicure.

Dental sealants—a thin plastic coating applied like nail polish by a dentist—are now recognized as the best way to prevent decay of the back teeth, according to the *Mayo Clinic Health Letter*.

A dentist first cleans and dries a patient's molars. Then he paints a clear or white-colored sealant onto them. The sealant hardens into a plastic shield preventing plaque from forming. Sealants will last about as long as fillings.

"Eighty percent of cavities occur on the chewing surface," the *Health Letter* says. Fluoride prevents cavities primarily on the non-chewing surfaces. Brushing, no matter how conscientious, cannot reach all food particles which find their way into the "pits" and "fissures" of the molars. Those food particles cause plaque.

Sealants are especially valuable for children.

They may assure that a child never has a tooth drilled. Sealants should be applied when molars first develop (around age six), the *Health Letter* says, and again when permanent teeth come in (about 11 or 12).

Children with badly positioned molars, and older or disabled persons may find sealants particularly helpful, the *Health Letter* adds.

Sealants were first introduced in the early 1970's and improvements have steadily been made since.

Although the American Dental Association thinks sealants should be an integral part of cavity control, especially in children, sealants are not widely used by dentists. But as a painless way to prevent cavities—and dental bills—sealants could make a lot of children and parents happy.

DEPRESSION

Depressed? Take a Cold Shower

For 15 years a 66-year-old Washington, D.C. woman suffered from depression. Every year when the weather turned warm the depression would begin. She experienced frequent crying spells, thoughts of suicide and social withdrawal. During a spring vacation in Florida one year, her depression began earlier. A summer vacation to cooler New England brought temporary remission.

Researchers are discovering that summer depression may be more common than winter depression. *The Journal of the American Medical Association* (JAMA) reports that depression and number of suicides reach a peak in late spring and summer.

Doctors Thomas A. Wehr, Norman Rosenthal and David A. Stack identified this patter of summer depression. They studied 12 patients who had suffered from chronic depression for many years, including the Washington D.C. woman. Nearly all reported a mood improvement following consistent exposure to lower temperatures, JAMA reports.

When the Washington D.C. woman was

confined to an air-conditioned house for five days and took regular 15-minute cold showers, her level of depression dropped dramatically, according to JAMA.

Such optimistic results have spurred National Institute of Mental Health investigators to plan a "larger controlled study of temperature therapy in summer depressives," JAMA reports.

Hope for Winter Depression

Who among us has not gone through the doldrums at some point during the months of January and February? With Christmas gone for another year and the gray, dreariness of winter seeming to last forever, we sometimes get depressed.

Psychiatrists have long recognized a link between clinical depression and winter. They call the phenomenon "seasonal affective disorder syndrome" or, more specifically, "recurring winter depression", according to the *Journal of the American Medical Association*.

"Daily exposure to extremely bright artificial lighting" has been the most successful treatment for recurring winter depression, says *Psychology Today*. Research now shows the treatment to be most effective in the morning.

Psychiatrist Alfred J. Lewy led a team of researchers who studied the effects of morning and evening light on eight winter-depressed people. The researchers had the eight patients, along with seven others not suffering from the disorder, sleep from 10 p.m to 6 a.m for four weeks. After one week, half were exposed to two hours of artificial bright light after awakening, the other half to the light two hours before bedtime. After one week the treatments were reversed. The last week everyone received the treatment both morning and evening.

The morning light treatment was found to be the most effective. Following the morning light exposure, the mood of the depressed people rose to almost the same levels they had experienced before the disorder. After the evening light treatment, however, their moods remained basically the same. When the two treatments were combined, moods improved "somewhat," *Psychology Today* reports, but not as much as they did with only morning light.

Lewy attributes the results to a hormone called melatonin, which fluctuates during the day. The researchers found the winter-depressed people secreted melatonin later in the evening than did the others. Morning light caused their bodies to produce melatonin at the normal time—early evening. Evening light, however, delayed production of the hormone, while both treatments produced melatonin at an intermediate hour.

Lewy concludes that consistent morning light appears to be an effective treatment for winter depression. He also believes, according to the *Psychology Today* article, the research may help in evaluating "other types of sleep and mood disorders" such as "shift work difficulties and jet lag."

Full Moon Blues

You may not feel compelled to howl at a full moon, but it could affect your mental and physical health more than you realize. Why?

The answer is not clear, but an increase in health problems does appear in thousands of people during this phase of the moon. Not only does the full moon seem to affect physical health, it affects mental outlook. Research indicates that more violent crimes are committed each month when the moon is full.

According to Dr. Ralph W. Morris, professor of pharmacology at the University of Illinois, blood pressure elevates, heart rates increase, bleeding ulcers can be more active, and chest pains can be more prevalent at the full moon. His hospital studies reveal that enzymes and many hormones are more active during a full moon, and body metabolism speeds up. Dr. Morris says other research shows that hemorrhaging can be more severe, stroke and epileptic convulsions can occur more often, and diabetics may experience more serious problems when the moon is full.

Dr. Morris admits that the reason the moon affects us physically has not been established but the alignment of the Earth, Moon and Sun and the electromagnetic and gravitational relationship of these celestial bodies may be the answer to the full moon blues our human bodies experience.

So what does all this moon madness have to do with your health? If you suffer from any of the above or other health problems, you may want to take extra precautions just before and during a full moon phase.

Eat right, exercise and get plenty of rest. If you are taking prescription medication be sure to follow your doctor's orders. If you are depressed easily or have frequent mood swings try relaxing more than usual. But don't worry, there is no evidence that you could turn into a werewolf during the next full moon.

Walk Away Depression

"Our young people are becoming less and less physically fit as we see more and more depressions and suicide," says Dennis Lobstein, Ph.D., a professor of exercise psychobiology and the director of the human performance laboratory at the University of New Mexico (reported in the *Medical Tribune*).

Lobstein sees a definite link between lack of exercise and depression in both young and old. U.J. Chodzko-Zajko, Ph.D., of The Center for Research on Aging at Purdue University, agrees that depression does not "automatically. . . increase with advancing age" but is associated with "things like reduced activity levels."

In his studies on the elderly, he found that high scores on the depression scale were found to be associated with low scores on the fitness scale. Mood changes occurred no matter how intense the activity, and Chodzko-Zajko believes even light calisthenics might have a significant beneficial effect in problems like depression in older people.

Lobstein's latest study compared ten joggers with ten sedentary middle-aged men. All were within the normal psychological range of depression (not pathological). It was found that exercise does decrease depression, according to the *Medical Tribune* article.

Also, the jogging group perceived themselves as having less stress then the sedentary group and had less "stress-circulating hormones" than the other men. Lobstein thinks this may be due to adaptations to long-term exercise training. "This affirms that depression is very sensitive to exercise and helps firm up a biochemical link between physical activity and depression," he concludes.

Depression Linked to Cancer Risk

A twenty-year study in Chicago recently revealed that men who experience depression are more likely to develop cancer, according to the *Harvard Medical School Mental Health Letter*.

In 1957, two thousand men who were 40 to 55 years old took a personality test. Among other things, the test included a depression scale which measured apathy, lack of self-esteem, sensitivity to criticism and unsociability.

The 210 men who developed cancer over the next 20 years had slightly, but significantly, higher than average scores on the depression scale, the *Letter* says. The men who scored higher on the scale were 1.4 times as likely to develop cancer and twice as likely to die of it.

The authors of the study think there might be either a "genetic tendency" or "something in their enviroment predisposing people to both depression and cancer. The researchers reported that depressed people may be more likely to die of cancer once they develop it because their immune systems are weakened.

DIABETES

Running Shoes May Prevent
Amputations in Diabetics

A side effect of diabetes is poor circulation, which sometimes leads to infection. In extreme cases gangrene sets in, forcing amputation. Five to fifteen percent of diabetics will undergo a leg amputation, according to *Prevention* magazine.

A little callus on the sole of the foot is often the cause of an amputation. The callus becomes ulcerated, infected and eventually gangrenous.

In a study by a foot doctor in Salt Lake City, "diabetes patients who wore running shoes for 18 months developed many fewer calluses than those patients who did not," *Prevention* reports.

Scott M. Soulier, D.P.M., M.S.P.H., of the Utah Diabetes Control Program, notes that most shoes, particularly those with leather bottoms, "do not really cushion the foot." He adds that "running shoes are specifically designed with extra cushioning that spreads pressure out over a larger area and helps prevent calluses."

His patients also prefer them to therapeutic shoes for less practical reasons: they look better.

New Treatment May Stop Diabetes

It appears a new drug, cyclosporine, may help prevent the most severe form of diabetes. Cyclosporine has previously been used to prevent rejection of transplanted organs. In a study conducted last year, half of a group of diabetics tested were able to discontinue using insulin after 60 to 90 days of cyclosporine treatment.

The diabetics studied suffered from Type 1, or juvenile diabetes. This is the most severe form, requiring daily insulin injections. Juvenile diabetes can lead to blindness, strokes and heart disease. In rare cases it may even cause death.

The Associated Press reported that low doses of this "transplant drug" appeared to reverse childhood diabetes, freeing youngsters from insulin injections. However, as promising as the new treatment may be, such a conclusion seems premature.

DIVERTICULITIS

A Diet To Help Control Diverticulitis

Diverticular disease is the out-ballooning of areas of the intestine into little pockets, in which fecal matter can lodge and cause infection. Many doctors who treat people with diverticular disease now recommend that they eat a diet which is high in dietary fiber or take a fiber supplement. The types of fiber recommended are the mushy types such as psyllium seed products or oat bran, as well as whole grain products. Hard types of fiber such as popcorn should be avoided.

People with diverticulosis or diverticulitis experience far fewer relapses if they consume appropriate dietary fiber daily, than if they eat a diet like the traditional American diet which is quite low in dietary fiber. Although the problems caused by diverticular disease will not disappear on a high fiber diet or after taking a fiber supplement daily, in most cases, they can be minimized and controlled so that surgery or antibiotic treatment can be avoided.

DIZZINESS

A Diet For Dizziness

Dizziness can be caused by your diet, according to Dr. Joel Lehrer at the New Jersey University of Medicine and Dentistry. About 90 percent of people who suffer from dizziness can be helped by a simple change in diet.

Some people's bodies don't properly absorb food, and this can cause dizziness, Dr. Lehrer explains. In a recent study, he found that changing the diet to 50 percent of calories from complex carbohydrates, like rice and spaghetti, 30 percent from fats, and just 20 percent from protein will reduce or eliminate dizziness in most people.

The amount of food and calories consumed should of course be based on the person's age, height, weight and body frame, but it's the breakdown of calories that is important. Changing to large amounts of complex carbohydrates, small amounts of lean meat and using only polyunsaturated fats may make a big difference in your life.

However, most diabetics and hypoglycemics will not be helped by this diet because their dizziness is not caused by their metabolism.

EAR PROBLEMS

A Better Solution to Ear Infections

Ear infections during childhood can lead to permanent hearing loss, yet many doctors and parents just treat them as everyday occurrences. Because they occur so frequently, it is easy to become lulled into using the same old treatment.

However, there is one type of infection-causing bacterium that has almost become resistant to most antibiotics. Branhamella catarrhalis, a bacterium also known as B-cat, resists most antibiotics, a fact that many doctors don't know, according to a recent survey by Dr. Manford Gooch from the University of Utah School of Medicine.

A couple of years ago, researchers determined that Augmentin® (amoxicillin and clavulanate) is more effective than Ceclor® (cefaclor) for treating most ear infections (*Journal of Pediatrics* 109:5,891). It is successful against the B-Cat bacterium in particular.

Dr. Gooch suggests that if ear infections do not start to improve after two days' treatment with antibiotics, parents should check with their children's doctors about trying Augmentin®.

EYESIGHT

This Eyesight Problem
May Be a Hidden Blessing!

If you are nearsighted you probably have above average intelligence, according to a study in *Clinical Genetics*. In a study involving over 2,500 children in California, children with IQ's over 135 were three times more likely to have shortsightedness, or myopia.

Myopia is an inherited trait. Based on survival of the fittest, the *Clinical Genetics* report believes that over the years shortsighted people who were less intelligent did not survive. Since only nearsighted people with high intelligence could endure primitive society, now myopia and intelligence are passed on together.

Nearsightedness can be easily corrected with concave lenses.

Over 65? Prevent Eyesight Deterioration

Dr. John Weiter of the Retina Foundation in Boston says that in people over 65 years of age deterioration of the retina (macular degeneration) is the leading cause of loss of eyesight.

Dr. Weiter adds that additional vitamin C, vitamin E and selenium can help prevent or reduce deterioration of the retina.

Take 50 micrograms of selenium daily, 400 International Units (I.U.'s) of vitamin E twice a day, and 500 milligrams of vitamin C per day, to help reduce retina damage, recommends Weiter. But first check with your doctor for his approval because large doses of vitamins and minerals may cause harmful side effects.

Better Lighting, Better Vision

Reduced vision in the elderly is sometimes related to poor lighting in their homes, according to an article in the *Lancet* journal. Researchers at St. Bartholomew's Hospital in London discovered that many elderly people used in their homes only one-tenth of the light that was used in the hospital. When the elderly people added a small light with a 60-watt bulb to illuminate their homes, vision improved in 82 percent of the patients.

Before loss of vision in elderly is assumed to be permanent, wattage in their home lighting should be checked.

This Vitamin Can Help Prevent Blindness

Your grandmother was right when she told you to eat your carrots because they're good for your eyes.

Yellow vegetables like carrots are high in Vitamin A. One early symptom of a Vitamin A deficiency is loss of vision in near darkness.

So to prevent night blindness, regularly eat vegetables high in Vitamin A.

Are You at Risk for Glaucoma?

Glaucoma is a disease of the eye that causes partial or complete loss of vision. Is it something you need to worry about?

If you are taking blood-pressure medicine or cortisone the answer is "yes," warns William R. Baldwin, Dean of the University of Houston College of Optometry.

Other people at high risk for glaucoma, who should be tested regularly, are those who have a family history of glaucoma and those who are black.

Once you reach 40, you should begin glaucoma tests every couple of years, even if you aren't in a high risk category, Baldwin recommends.

FATIGUE

A Mineral You May Be Missing

If you are getting adequate sleep each night but still fell "draggy," your body may be trying to tell you something. You may have an iron deficiency.

Unusual whiteness of the palms of the hands or the eyelids may be an early sign of iron deficiency. Lack of iron causes tiredness and is especially common in women. However, the *British Medical Journal* reports that tiredness is a symptom of advanced iron deficiency. If people with unusually pale palms or eyelids take iron supplements, a serious iron deficiency can be avoided. Women with heavy menstrual periods or those who are using intrauterine devices (IUDs) require more iron. Anyone who is suffering from fatigue may benefit from taking extra iron.

Whole-grain products, liver and organ meats, red meat, eggs, lima beans, prunes, spinach, raw broccoli, peas, fish and raisins are all good natural sources of iron. Iron supplements should be taken with food, orange juice or meals. Avoid taking iron supplements with tea, coffee or milk since they reduce its absorption.

Feeling Weak? You May Need
More of This Nutrient

Have you ever been so weak you had trouble just getting up in the morning? A woman recently felt that way and neither she nor her doctor could determine the reason.

Not until the woman was tested for deficiency of a certain mineral did the cause become apparent: her body was starved for potassium, a nutrient plentiful in bananas and oranges.

Millions of Americans are deficient in potassium. Among those at high risk are people like this woman who take diuretics for high blood pressure. While extracting salt and fluid from the body, diuretics can also remove potassium.

Lack of potassium manifests itself in tiredness and sluggishness, and causes leg cramps and irregular heartbeats.

The woman's doctor brought her potassium level back to normal with potassium supplements. Eating enough bananas and oranges should now maintain that level.

Pep Without Pills

Fatigue may be a symptom of a serious disease which needs medical treatment. A physician should be consulted if fatigue continues.

Fatigue may be caused by a deficiency of certain vitamins or minerals, including thiamine (vitamin B1), riboflavin (vitamin B2), niacin (vitamin B3), pantothenic acid (vitamin B5, vitamin B12, vitamin C or folic acid.

Over-consumption of caffeine may cause fatigue when the effects of the drug wear off, especially early in the morning. Monitor the number of caffeine-containing drinks (colas, coffee, tea) that you have daily, and start eliminating them.

Taking vitamin E in doses larger than the recommended daily dietary allowance (RDA) is reported to sometimes cause fatigue.

Taking extra vitamin C or the mineral manganese has been reported to reduce fatigue in some people.

FERTILITY

When Can a Middle-Aged Woman Stop Taking Contraceptives?

The oldest women to have a baby was Ruth Alice Kistler of Glendale, California, according to the *Guiness Book of Records*. In 1956, at the age of 57, she gave birth to a daughter.

This might lead a middle-aged woman to ask: "When is it safe to stop taking contraceptives?"

"It is often difficult to know when a woman has really stopped releasing an occasional ovum that could result in a mid-life pregnancy," *The Health Letter* says.

Nevertheless, the article suggests some steps you can take to avoid "unexpected blessings" during middle-age. First, a woman should wait at least twelve months after the last menstrual period before discontinuing the contraceptive. After that, if she has also gone through menopause, the chances of getting pregnant are quite slim. To be extra cautious, a woman may want to wait two years.

To determine if the menopause stage has begun or not, *The Health Letter* recommends blood tests to "evaluate hormone levels." Unfortunately these are not effective if a woman is using oral contraceptives. When temporarily off estrogen she may experience an "artificial menstrual period" and think wrongly she can still get pregnant, according to *The Health Letter*.

For those in doubt it may be wise to take another type of contraceptive for a time.

FOOD POISONING

How to Avoid "Stomach Flu"
Or Food Poisoning

What you assume to be stomach flu is probably food poisoning, says Patricia Long, salmonellae expert. Long says technically that there is no such thing as stomach flu. Usually the guilty organisms have entered your body through water or mishandled food.

The salmonellae bacteria "are the No. 1 cause of food-borne illness in the U.S.," Long says. She warns that "no turkey is fully cooked" and that too often chickens and turkeys are removed from the oven too soon and left to sit at room temperture This encourages bacteria to flourish and multiply like crazy.

Long notes that over one-quarter of the chickens consumed by Americans are contaminated with the salmonellae bacteria. Although 40,000 cases of salmonella food poisoning are reported each year, Long estimates as many as four million go unreported. "Most of these illnesses begin in our own kitchens," she says.

Common advice on how to avoid salmonella

includes not allowing frozen foods to thaw by leaving them outside the refrigerator or not leaving prepared foods out for over two hours.

Based on studies Long has conducted with the Infectious Disease Program of the University of California's School of Public Health, she discovered undercooked foul, particularly the stuffing in turkey, are rife with bacteria and multiply quickly when left outside the oven for long.

"Given the chance, salmonellae will live in almost anything edible," Long says, "but they prefer high-protein foods like meat and eggs. Foods with a lot of salt, sugar or acid, such as dry salami, jams, jellies, soy or citrus marinades and yogurt will slow down the bacteria from multiplying."

For example, Long says that contrary to popular belief, store-bought mayonnaise will not cause poisoning because it "has enough salt and acid to inhibit bacterial growth." Chocolate candy and milk, on the other hand, contain little salt or acid and will actually protect the bacteria from stomach acid.

Symptoms of salmonellae infection will occur within 12 to 48 hours and include nausea, diarrhea, abdominal cramps, fever and headache. Vomiting will occur on occasion.

Once you've got it, the best advice is to "drink fluids, stick to a bland diet and wait it out," Long says. Most have no idea it was salmonellae that hit them, unless the infection is severe enough to require a hospital visit. In such cases, "antibiotics may be prescribed to prevent bacterial invasion of the brain (meningitis), the lung (pneumonia) or the joints (arthritis)," Long reports. While these complications are rare, the Center for Disease Control in Atlanta estimates there are 500 to 1,000 deaths each year due to salmonellae poisoning.

Taking an antacid will allow bacteria though the stomach because stomach acid neutralizes it.

Long concludes the best prevention is to "assume that all meats are tainted, then prepare, cook and store foods with care," she says. Also, keep work spaces and sponges clean and watch out for microwave ovens. They often cook unevenly and bacteria may exist on uncooked portions of food.

FOOT PROBLEMS

Natural Care for Cold Feet

Cold feet may be a result of poor circulation caused by clogged arteries, heart problems, or stress Many people with diabetes, rheumatoid arthritis, collagen disease or lupus suffer from cold feet. Smokers often get cold feet because the effects of tar and nicotine in the tobacco cause the arteries to narrow and cause poor circulation. If you suspect that your cold feet are related to a circulation problem, you should discuss it with your doctor.

Simple exercise is the best way to warm up cold feet. Aerobic exercise, like walking, bicycling, swimming or jogging, is the best. With sustained aerobic exercise, the heart and blood vessels increase their tone. Circulation is improved, and, usually, the feet warm up. For an elderly person confined to bed or a chair, even rocking in a rocking chair can help improve circulation and warm up the extremities.

A warm or hot bath will raise body temperature and warm up the feet. If a bath is not practical, soak your feet in warm water. Placing a hot water bottle or an electric heating pad on the feet may also help. Do not get the water or heating pad too hot because the feet will not be sensitive, and you could burn yourself very easily.

Of course, wearing heavy socks or slippers is an easy way to keep the feet warm. Many people wear socks to bed because even blankets and comforters do not seem to keep their feet warm enough. Placing a blanket, quilt or afghan over the legs and feet while sitting is also effective. Many nursing home residents and people confined to a bed or a wheelchair use "lap quilts" to help keep their legs and feet comfortable.

Much Foot Surgery
A Thing of the Past with
These Home Remedies

If you're suffering from chronic pain in your heel and your doctor recommends surgery, *Prevention* magazine has a suggestion: get a second opinion.

Orthopedic doctors once thought chronic heel pain was a probable sign of calcium deposits called bone "spurs." Now they believe it is usually the result of tiny stress fractures.

The advent of new x-rays such as bone scans and tomography (or "depth" x-rays) offers doctors a more thorough basis on which to make a diagnosis, according to *Prevention*.

Doctor Charles Graham, of the University of Texas Health Science Center, says doctors now realize bone spurs don't normally cause pain nor are they serious enough to warrant removal.

Prevention magazine maintains that for stress fractures,"walking and stretching exercises and a heel pad in your shoe are all you need."

Unnecessary foot surgery, it is hoped, will now be a thing of the past.

GALL BLADDER DISEASE

Reduce Risk of Gallstones
While Preventing Heart Disease

If you reduce your risk of heart disease, chances are you won't be bothered by gallstones either. That's what Dr. Andrew Diel of the University of Texas Health Science Center in San Antonio says in a report from *Medical World News*.

"Heart disease and gallbladder disease share the same risk factors," the magazine explains. In other words, if you help prevent one disease, you help prevent both.

Diel's research of 2,990 people sought to determine how lifestyle affects the development of heart disease. The results confirmed findings of previous studies: "diabetes, high triglyceride levels, and a history of cigarette smoking are implicated in both heart disease and gall bladder disease."

"People with diabetes were diagnosed with gallstones twice as often as nondiabetics," Diel says. Twenty percent of those with high triglyceride levels were diagnosed as having gallstones and people who smoked were found to have gallstones more often than nonsmokers, Diel adds.

Preventing gallstones, Diel believes, is as easy (or hard) as preventing heart disease. He suggests consuming a moderate amount of alcohol (about three drinks a week) and maintaining a high level of the benefical HDL cholesterol. according to the *Medical World News* article.

GUM PROBLEMS

Before You See That
Surgeon . . . Try This

Oral surgery for gum disease is painful, expensive, and . . . necessary? Maybe not.

In fact, surgery may not be the best cure for gum disease, reports the *Journal of the American Dental Association*. Common gum disease is often treated with surgery that may not be necessary, says Dr. Sigurd Ramfijord, professor of oral surgery at the University of Michigan School of Dentistry.

In the journal Ramfijord explains that scaling at the gum line is just as productive as surgery. He recommends getting a second opinion before agreeing to oral surgery for common gum disease.

Homemade Toothpaste
Prevents Gum Disease

If you are bothered by gum disease or pyorrhea, you may want to make your own dentifrice from a simple salt solution.

Dr. Paul Keyes who has done work at the National Institute of Dental Research states that he has never seen a case of gum disease in a person who has regularly used salt or a soda dentifrice. He advocates brushing with a solution made by putting water in a glass and pouring enough salt in it so that no more will dissolve after stirring. Dr. Keyes states that his program is also good for treating early stages of pyorrhea.

Other dentists recommend brushing with baking soda; it also has a scouring effect that helps clean the gum line where gum disease and decay start around plaque that forms there. Be careful when following this advice. Excessive scouring can wear away tooth enamel and cause pain when drinking acidic beverages.

These natural cleansers may be just what the doctor ordered to help you keep your teeth.

HAIR LOSS

Hope For Ending Hair Loss

In the never-ending search for "eternal youth" everyone seems to be looking for a way to grow hair on bald heads or to prevent hair loss. A new drug (Rogaine®/minoxidil) that is rubbed into the scalp does help restore hair but not completely.

An even more hopeful treatment is still in experimental stages. Medical researchers in New Orleans have been combining minoxidil with tretinoin. Tretinoin is a prescription anti-acne medicine which is sold as Retin-A® and is a derivative of vitamin A. The new combination drug treatment seems to work better than minoxidil alone and provides hope for fewer bald heads in the future.

HEADACHES

Little-Known Causes
of Migraine Headaches
That You Can Easily Avoid

Do you suffer from occasional or chronic migraine headaches?

There's a good chance they can be avoided by eliminating particular foods from your diet, according to *Prevention* magazine.

A recent study, according to *Prevention* magazine, found allergies were responsible for migraine headaches in twenty-three of thirty-three sufferers. Each patient was allergic to an average of three foods. "Elimination of the guilty foods," *Prevention* reports, "brought headache relief, often within two weeks."

The offending foods included milk, cheese, eggs, chocolate, tea, tomatoes, coffee, shellfish, oranges, fish, wheat, rice and apples. Tyramine, the allergen in chocolate and "highly fermented cheese" is the most common culprit.

The researchers think headaches are probably triggered by "food substances causing sensitization of brain cells, which react to releasing histamine."

Understanding Your Headache

Headaches can be annoying and debilitating. To treat them effectively, it is important to know what kind of headache you are experiencing. According to Howard D. Hurland, M.D., author of *Quick Headache Relief Without Drugs*, these questions can help you evaluate your headache:

• *When did the headaches begin?* If they began suddenly, during a certain season of the year or while you were under some personal stress, it may be easy to pinpoint the type of headache you are experiencing. For example, a seasonal headache starting in the fall or spring could be an allergic reaction to pollen. Headaches that start during times of unusual stress could be tension headaches. These usually occur at the same time of day and are fairly constant.

• *What type of pain is the headache causing?* Some people have short bursts of sharp pain while others have a dull aching pain.

• *Where is the pain?* Is the pain centered in one area or one side of the head? If so, you may have a migraine headache.

• *Have the headaches progressed in severity?* Does it seem like the headaches are getting worse and worse? Headaches that start suddenly and continue to get more severe could be a warning sign of a brain tumor. If you get this kind of headache, you should contact your doctor at once.

• *When do they occur?* Is there a pattern to when you have them? For example, if you have them about four hours after eating, but they go away when you eat again, you may be suffering from low blood sugar. Just eating smaller, more frequent meals may help prevent this type of headache. Other headaches frequently are caused by eating certain foods. If you can keep track of when the headaches occur and how long they last, you may discover some food allergies that are causing the headaches. Are headaches a reaction to your emotions? Do you suffer from more headaches when you are angry or under stress?

• *Is any other part of your body affected by your headaches?* Problems with your sight, watery eyes or blurring associated with your headache may show that you are suffering from migraines. Sometimes sinus congestion can cause headaches. Check with your doctor for serious problems.

• *What other things seem to occur when you experience your headaches?* Many prescription and over-the-counter drugs can cause headaches as a side effect. Do you have headaches only when on a certain type of medication? Do they occur when you are outside? When you are under fluorescent lights? Do flashing lights bother you? Are they related to your menstrual cycle? Any circumstance that seems to trigger your headaches may provide clues to preventing the headaches.

• *Has anyone else in your family, like your mother or father, suffered from a similar type of headache?* Migraine headaches may be an inherited condition.

• *Does anything help relieve the pain?* If you take one aspirin or lie down and the pain goes away, it may be a very different kind of headache than one that requires a lot of painkillers.

• *Does anything seem to make the headache worse?* If you lie down and the headache seems to get worse, it could be a migraine headache. Headaches that are caused by brain tumors seem to get worse when the neck is constricted or during a sudden move, like a sneeze.

After you have narrowed down the type of headaches you experience you can deal more effectively with them. The following articles offer suggestions and help for the various types.

Natural Ways to Manage Your Migraine

People with migraine headaches should avoid

food containing tyramine. Tyramine dilates the blood vessels and contributes to causing many headaches. Avoid certain foods in the following groups because they contain high concentrations of tyramine:

- meat and fish — chicken livers, sausages, pickled herring, dried fish and beef
- dairy — aged cheese, sour cream and yogurt
- alcohol — red wine, champagne, sherry, beer, ale, Riesling and sauterne wines
- vegetables — sauerkraut and fava beans (broad Italian beans)
- flavorings — chocolate, soy sauce, vanilla, yeast and nitrites

Nitrates are also known to cause certain types of headaches. Watch for nitrate or nitrate additives on product package labeling. Be sure to avoid:

- hot dogs
- bacon
- sausage
- pepperoni
- salami
- ham
- all processed luncheon meats
- all cured meat

Many people have severe headaches after eating

food containing monosodium glutamate (MSG). MSG is often used in Chinese cooking, and these headaches and associated symptoms have been referred to as the Chinese Restaurant Syndrome. If you suffer from headaches after eating Chinese food, stop eating at Chinese restaurants or discuss with the chef the availability of MSG-free foods. MSG is also found in some meat tenderizers and prepared frozen dinners—be sure to read the labels.

Migraine headaches may be helped by resting quietly in a dark room for a couple of hours. Place a cool washcloth on your forehead. Make sure the cloth has been rinsed in cold water and wrung out. Or just sprinkle some water on your face before you lie down.

Dr. Seymour Diamond, director of the National Migraine Foundation, suggests placing an ice pack against your forehead or the pain's focal point. According to a recent study at the Diamond Headache Clinic, over 80 percent of migraine sufferers decided that the cold pack treatment helped reduce their headaches. Because a migraine headache is caused by the swelling of blood vessels, an ice pack may cause the blood vessels to return to a normal size, and the pain will cease, Diamond explains. For the best effect, he recommends placing the ice pack directly on the head and lying down for 30 minutes.

If it's not possible to lie down, try holding your hands under cold running water at a wash basin. This often provides some relief by causing the blood vessels in the hands to constrict, thereby affecting the body's vascular (blood vessel) system.

Physicians usually treat migraines with antihistamines, decongestants or caffeine and ergot-based drugs which constrict the enlarged blood vessels in the skull that cause migraines. If caffeine and ergot-based preparations don't work, physicians often prescribe beta-blockers or calcium channel blockers, drugs which are generally used as blood pressure reducers. Prescription drugs can cause severe side effects. Natural methods for treating migraines are preferred if they will work.

The most promising new natural treatment for migraines is to take magnesium supplements. Magnesium is usually deficient in the American diet, and magnesium supplements like magnesium chloride or dolomite, which is composed of calcium carbonate and magnesium carbonate, are quite helpful to many migraine sufferers, especially women who suffer from migraines during pregnancy or near the end of their monthly cycles.

Dietary Sweetener Causes Headaches

Studies have shown that diet "is an important element in the migraine headache process," according to the journal *Headache*. Chocolate, milk products, sherry and red wine have all been found to trigger migraine headaches, the journal says.

Evidence now suggests the popular dietary sweetener aspartame is the latest offender.

In a recent study at the University of Florida, aspartame was discovered to increase frequency of headaches, the journal reports.

A group of people suffering from periodic migraine headaches took a 300 mg. capsule of aspartame four times a day for four weeks. Another group ingested a placebo (a neutral pill containing no chemical). After a one-week "wash-out" period the subjects switched; the aspartame group now took the placebo. During the eight weeks, the subjects kept a record of their food intake and frequency of headaches, designating types (migraine, tension etc.) and how disabling they were.

The study concluded that "ingestion of aspartame by migraine sufferers may cause a significant increase in the frequency of migraines," according to the journal *Headache*. In addition, headaches were found to last a little longer when the subjects were taking aspartame, and several subjects had increased symptoms of dizziness, shaky feelings and poor vision during headaches. Aspartame was not found to increase the intensity of migraines, however.

The researchers note that with aspartame fast becoming the dietetic sweetener of choice in America, there are fewer and fewer products a migraine headache sufferer can safely use.

Stop Headaches Cold

Stop headaches simply by resting your head on a pillow? Yes, if the pillow happens to be a special ice pillow developed by Dr. Lee Kudrow, of the California Medical Clinic for Headache in Encino, California.

The horseshoe-shaped pillow has a pocket where a gel ice pack is inserted. When a person with a headache lies back on the pillow, the cold temperature causes muscles and arteries in the back of the head to contract, relieving pain.

The New England Center for Headache in Cos Cob, Connecticut, found that the pillows were effective for both tension and migraine headaches.

"As soon as patients felt the first dull pain they

were told to use the ice pillow," Dr. Sheftell, co-director of the Center, says. "It worked beautifully in four out of five cases."

In fact the patients were so satisfied with the pillows "they refused to give them back," Sheftell says.

Dr. Kudrow claims an 80 percent success rate with the hundreds of patients he has treated with his invention, named the "Suboccipital Ice Pillow."

He notes that the pillow is more effective than an ice pack because its horseshoe shape allows the cold to reach the muscles and arteries essential for headache relief. "It is also more comfortable," he adds.

Relax Your Headache Away

Is your headache the kind that drags on and on, constantly imparting a dull, steady pain? Then, you probably have a tension headache.

Usually, tension headaches are caused by stress or eyestrain. They may be helped by a simple massage of the scalp, neck and jaw area. Also, relaxation techniques, like taking a warm bath or listening to soft, calming music, may help. Refrain from all alcohol.

Caffeine: Friend or Foe in
Headache Relief?

Caffeine may provide relief from some people's headaches, but it can cause headaches in other people! How can this be?

According to Harold Gelb, D.M.D., in *Killing Pain Without Prescription*, drinking one or two cups of coffee may help constrict the blood vessels and reduce some people's headaches. However, constricting the blood vessels can cause headaches in other people, and withdrawing from habitual use of caffeine often causes headaches for a few days. Before you try coffee, tea, or other caffeine-containing products for headache relief, be sure you know if you are sensitive to caffeine.

HEARING LOSS

Little-Known Causes of Hearing Loss

Alcohol and sedative drugs can affect your hearing! By relaxing a certain muscle in the ear, alcohol and drugs reduce the natural protection against loud noises.

The way that it happens, explains the *Archives of Otolaryngology*, is that the ear muscle becomes relaxed, noises become magnified and the delicate eardrum may be damaged. The noise doesn't sound any louder, but the damage to the eardrum is increased.

Workers using loud equipment, like jackhammers or other power tools, and people listening to loud music need to be especially careful to avoid alcohol and drugs. The *Journal of the American Medical Association* (JAMA 258:35,13) also notes that noise in domed football stadiums can damage the hearing of the spectators.

As well as people who use alcohol and drugs, the journal reports that people with high blood pressure and those eating high fat foods, like fried chicken or hamburgers, experience increased noise damage.

Natural Help for Hearing Loss

In adults, particularly older adults, hearing loss may be the result of nerve damage. Zinc supplements have been shown, in many cases, to reverse a certain type of progressive inner ear nerve loss where people are deficient in zinc. It is also effective in some cases for people who suffer from ringing in the ears. In a recent study, fifty hearing loss patients with a confirmed zinc deficiency were given large doses of zinc, ten times the recommended daily dietary allowance.

All of the patients in this study experienced improvement in their hearing, and the ones who suffered from ringing in the ears also experienced improvement. Large doses of zinc like those used in this study should only be given upon a physician's advice because of the possibility of serious side effects.

HEART ATTACKS

Symptoms of a Heart Attack

Knowing the warning signs of a heart attack may save your life, especially if you do not delay in seeking medical help (see also "Emergency Musts for a Heart Attack Victim Who Is Alone").

Here are the symptoms of having a heart attack:

- heavy pressure or a choking or squeezing sensation in the center of the chest
- chest pain which may radiate down one or both arms, across the back, or up the neck
- shortness of breath
- an unexplained sensation or feeling of fear
- perspiration
- nausea
- dizziness or lightheadedness
- weakness or a fainting sensation
- angina pain that lasts for more than a few minutes or that doesn't go away upon administration of nitroglycerin and rest.

All of these symptoms need not be present to indicate that a heart attack is taking place. Some can be caused by other problems, like indigestion. Some heart attacks are called silent heart attacks, because there is not any advance warning. But many heart attacks can be partially anticipated, because the victim has suffered, perhaps for years, from angina pectoris or heart problems.

Emergency Musts For a Heart Attack Victim Who Is Alone

There is nothing more frightening than facing a life-and-death situation alone. Knowing what to do can give you the confidence you need to act promptly and save your own life.

If you are experiencing one of the warning signs of a heart attack (see "Symptoms of a Heart Attack"), you should first of all realize that within ten seconds after the heart stops beating, a victim will become unconscious. If someone else is around, and they know CPR (cardiopulmonary resuscitation) they can help keep oxygen flowing to the brain until medical aid arrives. However, if you are alone it is difficult to keep the oxygen flowing. Deep coughing and deep breathing may be your only hope, reports *Emergency Medicine*.

Take a deep breath, then cough long and hard, like you are trying to remove phlegm from the chest. The coughing helps to stimulate the heart and keep blood flowing, while the deep breaths help provide oxygen to the brain. Coughing and deep breathing may help for only a few minutes, but this may allow you enough time to get to a phone for emergency help. Alternating deep breaths and deep coughs must be continued every two seconds until regular heartbeats begin.

Most heart attack victims who make it to the hospital will survive, but unfortunately victims usually wait many hours before seeking medical help. Most people who die of heart attacks die outside the hospital. Knowledge of the symptoms of a heart attack and prompt action by calling an ambulance for a quick trip to the hospital can make the difference between life and death for a heart attack victim.

Something From Your Medicine Chest May Prevent A Heart Attack

You've taken aspirin to get rid of your headache, but did you know it may keep a heart attack away as well?

That's right, according to the *New England Journal of Medicine* (318:4, 262-264). The research showed that an aspirin every other day would reduce the risk of heart attack *by one half* compared to people not taking aspirin. Although the study was scheduled for two more years, the researchers decided to publish their preliminary results because they felt that so many lives could be saved. Since people without previous history of heart disease were used in the study, almost everyone can benefit from the results. However, the researchers stress that no one should start aspirin therapy without his doctor's knowledge and consent.

Buffered aspirin (325 milligrams) was used in the study, but regular aspirin or enteric coated aspirin would also be effective, the researchers say. However, acetaminophen (like Tylenol®) does not have the same effect. Ibuprofen (like Advil® and Nuprin®) was not included in this study, but it may also help reduce blood clots leading to heart attacks. The researchers tested several different doses of aspirin and found that one aspirin every second day was the most effective. An aspirin every day (for people without previous heart problems) did not increase its protective effect but did increase unwanted side effects like stomach bleeding and indigestion.

It is important to remember that in healthy people and heart patients, aspirin therapy does *not* treat the plaque and artery disease that causes heart attacks. Aspirin only reduces the blood's ability to clot. So all known ways of fighting artery disease (atherosclerosis) like not smoking, reducing fat intake, lowering high blood pressure and exercising, should be carefully followed.

If you have already suffered from a heart attack, the research on aspirin may be even more valuable. The Food and Drug Administrtion (FDA) announced that heart patients can reduce the chance of having another heart attack by taking an aspirin each day. For men who have already had heart attacks, one aspirin tablet per day can cut their risk of heart attack by twenty percent. Men with unstable angina (chest pains) who take daily aspirin will reduce their risk of recurring angina by up to fifty percent.

Aspirin inhibits the action of small cell fragments in the blood, called platelets, which have a role in blood clotting. In this way, aspirin is thought to decrease the likelihood of having a heart attack, since a heart attack usually results when a clot blocks the blood flow to the heart muscle.

However, aspirin should not be used as a substitute for other preventative therapies for heart attacks, cautions FDA commissioner Frank E. Young, M.D. People with a history of ulcers, certain types of strokes, stomach bleeding, or kidney or liver disease should not take aspirin.

Doctors at the Sarasota Retina Institute also report that aspirin causes an increased risk of blindness due to bleeding in the retina (*New England Journal of Medicine* 318:17, 1126). James D. Kingham, M.D. warns that the availability of aspirin and the increased feelings that aspirin is safe may "usher in a new wave of blindness." Anyone with sight problems, especially the aging, should not take aspirin without their doctor and ophthalmologist's knowledge and monitoring.

How You Can Help Your Loved One Recover From A Heart Attack

Recovering from a heart attack can be difficult especially when a spouse is worried about your every move.

Researchers at Stanford University tried an experiment that allowed the spouse to participate in the physical therapy of the heart attack victim. Not only did they watch the activities, they felt compelled to perform the same treadmill stress tests, side-by-side with their spouses. According to an article in *Body Bulletin*, the loving spouses could see and experience the physical activity and stress of the treadmill.

Once they saw how the heart attack victim had endured the exercise, they didn't worry about them as much at home during their recovery. They encouraged their partners and were more tolerant of their activities. By having a spouse's support, recovery was less stressful and a little easier for the heart attack victim.

Your Eyelids May Warn You of a Heart Attack

You may know that high blood cholesterol levels increase the risk of heart attack. But did you know your eyelids can tip you off to that danger?

Soft, yellowish patches around the eye, particularly on the eyelids, may signal an elevated cholesterol level, the *Mayo Clinic Health Letter* reports. These patches of skin are called xanthelasma. People with the condition are often unaware of its significance.

If you notice the little folds of skin developing, it is an indication that you should take some steps to lower blood cholesterol levels and prevent a heart attack.

First you should lower your blood pressure and begin exercising on a regular basis. Also, maintain a diet low in saturated fats and cholesterol, and try to get down to your ideal body weight.

Xanthelasma won't always be present where there are high blood cholesterol levels. But if you notice the yellowish patches on your eyelids, they are a warning to do something about high cholesterol before it's too late.

HEART PROBLEMS

High Risk Factors For Heart Disease

The more risk factors for heart disease that you have, the more careful you must be about working to maintain a healthy-heart life style. These risk factors are beyond our control:

- a personal history of heart problems or stroke
- an immediate family member who has had a heart attack, sudden death or stroke, especially before they were 65
- being male
- being diabetic

On the other hand, there are some risk factors that can be reduced. The following are up to you:

- smoking
- being more than 30 percent over your ideal weight
- not exercising regularly
- a cholesterol level over 200, especially if it's higher than 240
- high blood pressure

Many of these factors that we can control we covered in separate sections of this book. Be sure to study those articles carefully, and give your heart—and life—a chance!

Natural Ways to Fight
Coronary Heart Disease

Many researchers recommend the following natural methods for treating or reducing the chances of developing coronary heart disease (or coronary artery disease):

• *Reduce the Amount of Fat in the Diet.* Especially reduce saturated fats which are usually found in meat and dairy products. The American Heart Association recommends that saturated fats comprise only 30 percent of total calorie intake; others suggest even lower levels of from only 10-15 percent. These levels are substantially lower than the levels found in typical American diets. In a simplified form they mean eating less meat, dairy products, eggs and other sources of saturated fats and cholesterol, while relying more on starches and low-fat sources of protein such as broiled fish and poultry.

Diets high in protein, as from meat, and low in lysine, as from low-fat dairy products, can contribute to heart disease.

• *Lower Blood Cholesterol.* High levels of cholesterol in the blood are a risk factor for coronary heart disease. It's a good precaution to measure cholesterol and its HDL (high-density lipoprotein) and LDL (low-density lipoprotein) fractions every time blood is drawn for a physical exam. High LDL levels are harmful, but high HDL levels can help prevent coronary heart disease. See "Tips for Reducing Cholesterol."

• *Gradually Lose Weight.* People who are overweight need to gradually lose weight until normal weight levels are reached and maintained. The heavier an obese person is, the more likely he is to have a heart attack. Excess pounds put extra strain on the heart.

• *Do Not Smoke.* Quit smoking to reduce chances of heart disease. Heavy cigarette smokers have twice the death rate from coronary heart disease as non-smokers. Non-smokers who live in the same house with a heavy cigarette smoker have higher death rates from coronary heart disease than non-smokers who do not live with a person who smokes. Heavy cigarette smokers have a life expectancy as much as ten years less than that of non-smokers.

• *Get Moderate Physical Exercise.* Brisk walking is the type of exercise recommended by most doctors. It's preferred because it puts a moderate amount of stress on the heart and lungs and serves to strengthen them, while not exerting them to the point where it's likely that a heart attack would occur.

A recent study shows that older people with painful foot problems, which prevented normal standing or walking activities, had extremely high rates of heart attacks—several times higher than expected.

It's a paradox that while many studies show that regular, sustained aerobic exercise strengthens the heart, helps the circulation, and is a positive benefit, they also indicate that sudden, unaccustomed bursts of exercise can lead to heart attacks in susceptible people.

• *Avoid Stressful Situations*. Avoid pressure in the office. Steer clear of arguments and heavy strenuous exercise like shoveling snow.

• *Lower High Blood Pressure*. Reducing high blood pressure helps lessen the chance of developing coronary artery disease.

• *Doctor-Prescribed Aspirin*. Aspirin is thought to decrease the likelihood of having a heart attack. See the article "Something From Your Medicine Chest May Prevent a Heart Attack."

• *Avoid Alcohol*. Alcoholism or heavy consumption of alcoholic beverages is a definite risk factor which leads to increased rates of heart attacks.

- *Eat Salt Water Fish.* The oil found in some fresh water fish and all salt water fish has recently been discovered to be beneficial in raising HDL levels in the blood. Recent population studies show that people who eat substantial amounts of cold water fish like trout, salmon, mackerel or cod have lower rates of coronary heart disease than other people, even if the total amount of fat in the diet remains about the same. These new studies suggest that the addition of fish to the diet, and especially the replacement of much red meat and dairy products with fish, could reduce the chance of developing coronary heart disease.

- *Pay Attention To Heredity.* People whose parents or other close relatives have had coronary heart disease are at greater risk than people who come from families with low rates of coronary heart disease. Although heredity is not controllable, the presence of coronary heart disease in close family members is a risk factor which indicates that it is more likely to develop; all possible precautions should be taken.

- *Vitamins and Minerals.* See "Vitamins And Minerals That Help Your Heart."

- *Estrogen for Women during Mid-life and Menopause.*

- *Avoid Areas of Air Pollution.* Ozone,

163

sulfur dioxide, nitrogen dioxide, cigarette smoke, carbon monoxide, hydrocarbons, nitrogen oxide and photochemical substances are air pollutants that can worsen heart problems.

• *Avoid Sudden Changes to High Altitude.* Living at high altitudes may not be as harmful to the heart as has been thought. In the past, doctors thought that high altitudes caused heart problems. However, new research by the American Heart Association shows that the opposite may be true. James K. Alexander, M.D., of Baylor College of Medicine in Houston participated in the study called "Operation Everest Two." Over a 40-day span, seven men were put into a low-pressure chamber that simulated the effects of 29,000 feet altitude. Dr. Alexander said they were surprised to discover that the heart actually seemed to do better at high altitude! In spite of this study, sudden changes to high altitudes should be avoided, and people with severe heart disease may be helped by moving to low altitudes. Ask your physician for his advice.

Self-treatment, especially in the case of a serious illness like coronary artery disease, is not a good idea. Even though natural methods of preventing coronary artery disease may be helpful, there is no substitute for the care of a skilled physician if you already have coronary artery disease or if you ever had a heart attack.

Please consult your physician before changing any established treatment program for coronary heart disease.

Test Gives Early Warning of Heart Disease Risk

We can reduce our chances of contracting hypertension and atherosclerosis but once symptoms of those illnesses appear, it may already be too late.

A new genetic screening test, however, may eventually make it possible to identify persons at risk for atherosclerosis or hypertension before clinical signs of disease appear, the *Medical World News* reports.

Researchers in California and a Michigan researcher have discovered "genetic markers," which signal "increased risk for atherosclerosis and hypertension, "the article says.

Because atherosclerosis can be caused by a defect in any one of a number of genes, developing a genetic test for it is not easy, notes Dr. Phillipe Frossard, project director at California Biotechnology. He believes the screening test will probably involve "an array of markers that in various combinations may produce disease," according to *Medical World News.*

Frossard has identified fourteen markers for hypertension so far, focusing on genes involved with regulating blood pressure. A link between the markers and hypertension is being studied in 70 hypertension patients and 30 not so afflicted at Cornell University Medical Center.

Frossard believes that genetic testing to predict hypertension and atherosclerosis in those with no symptoms will become routine within a year or two.

Not only will accurate prediction of hypertension and atherosclerosis enable doctors to truly "practice preventive medicine," Frossard says, but also the prescribed treatment will be more effective if the doctor knows "what genetic defect is causing the problem."

HEART WELLNESS

Vitamins and Minerals
That Help Your Heart

In addition to the well-known therapies for preventing heart problems, here are some facts you should know about how specific vitamins and minerals affect your heart.

A pyridoxine (vitamin B6) deficiency may contribute to coronary heart disease. Pyridoxine supplementation may be especially helpful in preventing heart and artery disease for people who eat high-protein diets. When meat is cooked, it loses much of its pyridoxine, which could have been used by the body to help break down by-products of methionine, one of the amino acids found in protein. By-products of methionine are thought to damage the arteries and cause heart disease much like the process which is involved to a much greater extent in homocystinuria (an hereditary enzyme-deficiency disease). Taking supplements of small amounts of pyridoxine with each meal containing cooked meat may help to prevent some coronary heart disease.

A magnesium or selenium deficiency may result in coronary heart disease. People living in areas where these minerals are deficient in the water supply have high rates of heart disease.

When niacin (vitamin B3) is taken in high dosages, it has been shown to reduce the amount of cholesterol in the blood *(Journal of the American Medical Association)*. In a study of heart attack victims, it was found that people who took high doses of niacin had an eleven percent lower death rate than those who did not.

Niacin must be administered in high doses to be effective against heart disease and cholesterol. But, because of the significant side effects of large doses of niacin, it should be taken only under a doctor's supervision. Some people, such as those with high blood pressure, diabetes, gout or ulcers, should not take niacin at all. The niacinamide form of the vitamin should not be used because it does not lower blood fats by a significant amount.

Food sources for niacin include yeast, fish, poultry, liver, meat, whole-grain products (except corn which contains an inactive form of niacin), peanuts, potatoes, beans and mushrooms.

People receiving digitalis or other heart medication should not take calcium ascorbate (a vitamin C formulation) since irregular heartbeats may occur.

Studies by Kurt A. Oster, M. D., and others indicate that folic acid may be helpful in the treatment and prevention of heart disease. Larger, controlled studies are necessary to confirm these studies.

Another medical doctor states that folic acid may stop the progress of coronary heart disease by neutralizing xanthine oxidase, an enzyme found in milk fat that may be harmful to the arteries, and by restoring a substance which repairs damage to arteries and helps stop the fatty buildup which is found in hardening of the arteries.

Does Your Hair Affect Your Heart?

How does the amount of hair you have affect your heart? Well, doctors aren't quite sure, but men with hair on their ears develop heart disease more often than men with "hairless" ears.

Researchers at Nassau Hospital in New York speculate that the amount of testosterone, the male hormone, may affect both the incidence of having hairy ears and the rate of heart problems.

Even though most men (about seventy-five percent) have hairy ears, the researchers recommend that all men with this characteristic lower their cholesterol, lose weight and exercise.

169

Surgery, Safety, And Your Heart

Avoid heart catheterization for diagnostic purposes until its safety record has been confirmed, doctors warn in the journal *Chest*. About one-fifth of heart attack victims have their hearts catheterized to help determine blood pressure and flow.

A long flexible tube is inserted in a vein and pushed through the heart to the lung. Although the catheter provides the doctor with valuable information, researchers at the University of Massachusetts Medical School discovered that between ten and fifteen thousand deaths each year seemed to be caused by using the catheter. The researchers believe that catheterization definitely involves risks, and yet it is often used unnecessarily. Other doctors suggest that the death rate is high because most people who receive the treatment are in "worse shape" than patients who don't receive catheterization. However, even with the variations in health, using the catheter seems to increase the risk of death.

Blood-thinning heparin may be given during routine surgery to help reduce blood clots, announced the *New England Journal of Medicine* (318:17). Blood clots can lead to heart attacks, strokes or blood clots in the lung and are considered a dangerous possibility following surgery. Researchers in Oxford, England, found that giving heparin during surgery cut the death rate from surgery-related clots by half.

It May Be Possible to Extend Your Heartbeats for an Extra Twenty-Four Years

Is it possible to literally "run your heart out"? Researchers at Cleveland Clinic Foundation and Case Western Reserve University School of Medicine decided to find out, reports the *New England Journal of Medicine.*

Recent studies have focused on the "cardiovascular risks" of running, not just the musculo-skeletal, the *Journal* says. The studies reflect new skepticism about the ultimate worth of pounding the ground all those miles to the heart of runners.

One group of skeptics say the few years runners add to their lives are spent running. Another theory states: "You only get so many total heartbeats, and when you exhaust this allotment you die."

To evaluate those claims, the researchers employed a discipline more exacting than science.

They relied on the concepts of mathematics.

They first multiplied the average human heartbeat of seventy-two beats per minute by an ordinary life expectancy of seventy five years, to arrive at the "total human heartbeat allotment." Although the average runner's heart rate increases more than threefold when he runs (up to one hundred eighty beats per minute), his resting pulse is usually 23.6 percent slower than the average person's, the *Journal* says. Since his heart beats slower most of the time, it would take him 99.4 years to use up the total human heartbeat allotment the researchers figure.

By the finite heartbeat theory, all other things being equal, a runner would live 24 years more than a non-runner. (The researchers assumed that the runner ran five times a week, which adds up to 0.915 years of total running time.)

"The life extension of 24.4 years suggests that running is an efficient way of reallocating heartbeats," the researchers state. The calculations, they believe, unequivocally "support the benefits of regular conditioning." However, in our opinion, their conclusions are dependent upon a shaky, unproven assumption. They assume that we only have a quota of heartbeats in our lifetime.

Change of Heart Comes with Change of Life?

For years women have used estrogen replacement to help them through menopause. Now it appears estrogen may be equally valuable to the heart, according to *Prevention* magazine.

Researchers lead by Dr. Graham Colditz studied 120,000 women and found that postmenopausal women who take estrogen have about half the risk of having a heart attack as those who don't take it.

A more recent study revealed that women who had both ovaries removed before menopause and did not take estrogen replacement had double the risk of heart disease as those who took estrogen after surgery, *Prevention* reports.

Dr. Colditz says this study confirms the estrogen/heart disease association noticed in previous studies.

Colditz attributes the benefits of estrogens to an ability to raise HDL (beneficial) cholesterol levels and lower LDL (artery clogging) levels.

The benefits are so marked, Colditz believes, that estrogen-replacement therapy should be considered "at this stage if the benefits outweigh the risks."

HEMORRHOIDS

Rubber Bands Instead of Surgery?

Hemorrhoids are enlarged, dilated veins of the rectal and anal passages. They can occur at any age, but they are found more often as people age.

Surgery is often recommended for severe hemorrhoids, but "banding" the hemorrhoids is very effective, less painful, and can be done in a clinic. It is usually much less expensive than surgery. Instead of completely cutting out the hemmorrhoid, a rubber band is tightly placed around the root. Within a few days the blood supply to the hemorrhoid will be stopped and the dead hemorrhoid will dry up and fall off.

Because banding avoids surgery, there are usually fewer complications. With a 92 percent success rate for banding compared to a 95 percent success rate for surgical removal, banding is a good alternative to surgery, the *Archives of Surgery* reports.

Electric Current Treatment, Alternative to Hemorrhoid Surgery

Ineffective treatments for hemorrhoids have

been around since the day of the ancient Greek father of all doctors, Hippocrates. He dealt with hemorrhoids by burning them off with a red hot poker, according to *The Health Letter*. Unfortunately, recovering from hemorrhoid surgery today is just about as painful.

A new non-surgical treatment for the age-old malady may finally work well without the painful side-effects. Dr. Daniel Norman of the University of Nevada School of Medicine claims a one hundred percent success rate using electric current, *The Health Letter* reports.

Norman gave 42 hemorrhoid patients an average of two to three treatments. "He reportedly eliminated all the hemorrhoidal tissue, and the patients were symptom-free 18 months later," the article states. Mild hemorrhoids required a mere six minutes of the smallest amount of current. Grade four (the most severe) hemorrhoids needed twice the current for eight to nine minutes each treatment. The hemorrhoidal tissue came off in three to ten days leaving the normal tissue apparently undamaged.

According to Dr. Norman, this technique has been effective on hemorrhoid patients that have not been successfully treated with surgery.

However, the *Letter* cautions that further

studies must be done to substantiate Dr. Norman's results.

Past techniques like freezing hemorrhoids, for instance, could not eliminate enough harmful tissue without destroying normal tissue. The effectiveness and apparent harmlessness of Dr. Norman's treatment need further verification.

HICCUPS

Something New To Try For Hiccups

You've become so annoyed by an attack of hiccups, you're ready to try anything, right?

Well, here's another home remedy to add to your list of cures for hiccups. Try sucking on a wedge of lemon. Many singers use lemons to help clear their throats, so maybe that's related to how the powerful lemon works against hiccups.

IMMUNE SYSTEM

Natural Ways To Avoid Getting Sick

There are several things you can do to help keep your immune system working at its best to increase your body's ability to fight off disease.

• *Use your nose.* By breathing through your nose rather than through your mouth, you allow the tiny nose-hairs to filter the air and provide protection against some of the billions of particles transmitted through the air.

• *Don't smoke.* Keep your "filtering system" in top condition. Smoking damages your lungs (which causes lowered immunity) and smoking also damages the protective hairs in the breathing passages.

• *Allow for rest and relaxation.* Don't be afraid to pull back and take some time for yourself. Be sure to include some quiet time since noise lowers your immunity level.

• *Get adequate sleep.* Each adult requires a different amount of sleep. Be sure to know what your daily requirements are and allow your body to re-energize itself daily. Lack of sleep is known to make us more susceptible to infections, stress and flare-ups of chronic illnesses.

Laugh Poor Health Away—It Works

Research has shown that the body's immune system is weakened by stress and depression. Now it appears that even temporary mood swings may affect the ability of the body to fight off sickness.

Psychologist Arthur A. Stone and a group of researchers studied 30 dental students to determine the effect of minor stress on the immune system. The men were given "an unfamiliar but harmless protein" for a little over two months, *Psychology Today* reports. The levels of antibodies their bodies produced against it (the process by which the immune system fights viruses) were traced. The students also reported three times a week on their moods.

"Good moods corresponded to a bolstered immune response, better enabling the body to 'reject' the substance," *Psychology Today* reports. On the other hand, bad moods and low production of antibodies were found to occur on the same day.

" Minor, daily mood fluctuations are associated with immune functioning," the researchers concluded. While past studies merely linked stress to sickness, now it appears, as *Psychology Today* says, "happiness may play a part in keeping people healthy."

Zinc Intake Builds Immune System

A relationship between low zinc levels and weak "immune response" in older people has been discovered by researchers at the New Jersey Medical School in Newark, according to *Prevention* magazine.

The researchers found that most older people do not receive an adequate amount of zinc. Ninety percent of those studied were getting less than the Recommended Dietary Allowance (RDA) of 15 milligrams a day, the researchers say.

"Our data suggests that zinc supplementation may enhance immune functions in the elderly," they report.

These conclusions support the findings of studies on zinc deficiency in animals. The *British Journal of Medicine* reports that low zinc levels in animals during pregnancy can cause "immune dysfunction persisting for several generations."

Nutrition Reviews cites the example of Holstein-Friesan cattle with severe zinc deficiencies caused by a "genetic mutation" which inhibits zinc absorption. As a result of the low zinc levels, the cattle suffer from an immune deficiency disease which leaves them susceptible to disease-causing organisms.

Nutrition Reviews notes that children can be cured of the hereditary desease acrodermatitis enteropathica with zinc supplements.

Researchers have also found that lack of adequate zinc can produce profound immune deficiencies in those with "protein-calorie malnutrition, advanced cancer, trauma, and sickle cell anemia," *Nutrition Reviews* says. By taking dietary zinc supplements, these problems can be fought, and perhaps corrected, through a stronger immune system.

IMPOTENCE

Natural Ways of Combating Impotence

Impotence usually occurs for physical reasons and not psychological reasons. It occurs more often as people get older.

Taking vitamin E has been advocated by some to increase sexual function and to combat impotence. Vitamin E is proven to increase fertility in some people, but there is no evidence that it increases sexual drive or reduces impotence. As a matter of fact, one study showed that *taking large doses of vitamin E may cause reduced sexual function.*

Taking zinc supplements has been reported to improve some cases of impotence, but its effectiveness is unproven. Large doses of zinc supplements can be dangerous, so any zinc supplementation should be within the recommended daily dietary allowance (15 mg. per day for adults).

Good overall health is the best way to combat many cases of impotence. Regular, daily exercise, keeping weight under control and eating a healthy diet with lots of whole grain products and little fat can improve overall health and perhaps, in some cases, counteract a tendency towards impotence.

A mild stimulant like caffeine in coffee sometimes will help reduce impotence.

Drinking alcohol even in small amounts is a widespread cause of impotence. Many people can reverse impotence immediately by giving up alcohol.

Smokers have higher rates of impotence than non smokers.

Prescription Drugs
That Can Cause Impotence

Prescription drugs for high blood pressure and ulcers can cause impotence, warns Dr. William Masters, of the Masters and Johnson Institute in St. Louis. A decrease in sexual desire or impotence is a well-known side effect of many drugs often prescribed for older men, Masters says.

According to *Drug Interactions and Side Effects Index*™ of the *Physicians Desk Reference*, impotence is listed as a side effect of over one hundred prescription drugs. Diuretics, used to treat high blood pressure, and anti-ulcer drugs like Tagamet® and Zantac® are some of the most widely-used drugs that cause impotence.

If you suspect that your medications are causing

impotence problems, do *not* alter your medication. Talk to your doctor about changing to a different drug with less bothersome side effects.

INCONTINENCE

A Prescription Drug May Be Responsible

Incontinence is a problem at any age, but many people over 65 just consider it a normal part of growing old. However, incontinence can be the side effect of a prescription drug.

Some of the drugs that may be responsible are: Etrafon®, Halcion®, Mellaril®, Octamide®, Permitil®, Protostat®, Reglan®, Serax®, Serentil®, Triavil®, Valium® and Xanax®. If you have poor bladder control and take one of the above listed drugs, talk to your doctor. Do *not* stop taking or alter your medication without consulting your doctor.

INDIGESTION

Old-Fashioned Candy Relieves Gas

An old-time favorite candy, peppermint, may relieve stomach gas. Thomas L. Kun, a California gastroenterologist disclosed in *Prevention* magazine recently that peppermint helps to release intestinal gas.

Peppermint allows the sphincter muscle at the base of the esophagus to relax, and as this happens stomach gas is released. If someone swallows a lot of air when he eats and he feels bloated, relaxing this muscle will relieve his indigestion.

Taking eight drops of spirit of peppermint (available from your pharmacist) in warm water, drinking peppermint tea made from real peppermint leaves, or eating mints made with genuine oil of peppermint are good sources of peppermint recommended by this gastric specialist.

One word of caution is given about this remedy: If you have a tendency toward heartburn, you should avoid this treatment. It may mean your sphincter muscle is so weak that it is allowing acid out of your stomach. In this case, the sphincter muscle should remain as tense as possible, so you should avoid peppermint.

INFERTILITY

A Simple Procedure
That Can Give You Hope

Many women suffer from "tubal infertility," caused when the fertilized egg cannot get through the fallopian tube into the womb. If a tubal blockage was caused by scar tissue or other material, the only way to solve the block has been to undergo expensive surgery.

Now there is a simple new technique that can restore fertitily in women without surgery. This new technique, being tested at Oregon Health Sciences University, uses a catheter that is inserted through the vagina and the womb into the blocked fallopian tube. Once the blockage is reached the doctor uses a small wire-like tube to break up the problem. This opens the fallopian tube enough for a fertilized egg to pass through.

The technique is similar to the use of catheters to help open blocked arteries in the heart.

INSOMNIA

Sleeping without Sedatives

Did you know that commonly prescribed drugs, stimulants and stressful lifestyles can cause insomnia? Here are some of the usual causes of sleeplessness, cited by the *Harvard Medical School Health Letter*:

• lack of routine sleeping habits, especially inconsistent bedtimes or waking times

• an emotional crisis, such as work-related problems, loss of money or marital problems

• being overaroused. Worrying about tomorrow's activities or planning events while trying to sleep is not productive. Perfectionists often suffer from this type of insomnia because they keep reviewing details in their mind, rather than relaxing and preparing for sleep.

• lack of exercise or daily activities. Unemployment or physical infirmities may limit daily activities.

• caffeine. Avoid all sources including coffee, tea, chocolate, soft drinks, diet pills and some prescriptions and over-the-counter drugs. A s k your pharmacist for a complete list of drugs that contain caffeine.

- developing a tolerance to sleeping pills
- alcohol. It is common to awaken in the middle of the night after drinking alcohol.
- over-the-counter diet pills (most contain stimulants)
- certain prescription drugs including:
  - -asthma drugs
  - -blood-pressure reducing drugs
  - -heart-rhythm regulating drugs (anti-arrhythmics)
  - -hormones, like estrogen, progestin, oral contraceptives, and adrenal hormones
  - -steroids
  - -levodopa and other drugs used to treat Parkinson's disease
- being bored or lacking a purpose in life
- depression
- naps taken during day
- snoring or other breathing problems that interrup normal sleep
- nervous system diseases affecting the brain, spinal cord or nerves
- severe pain, fever or itching that disturbs sleep
- gland problems involving the thyroid gland, parathyroid gland, ovaries, testes, pituitary gland, adrenal gland or the pancreas

- illegal drugs like marijuana or cocaine

Here are some suggestions to help you sleep before you reach for a sedative:

- Fresh air in the bedroom may help alleviate insommnia. Opening the windows wide for about 10 minutes, then leaving them open about an inch can provide a good supply of oxygen and fresh air for the night's sleep. A stuffy room may inhibit your ability to sleep, according to Dr. Charles Wolfe, Jr., of the Sleep Disorder Center in Chicago, Illinois.

- Creating your personal perfect environment for sleeping can be helpful, according to the *Mayo Clinic Health Letter*. Fresh air, a cool room temperature, total darkness, quietness, and clean bedsheets may help you get a good night's sleep.

- If you are in a situation where complete silence is impossible to achieve, try masking the sounds. A small air-conditioning unit, a fan, a stereo or a radio set at low volume may block out annoying sounds and create a monotonous environment for sleeping.

- Don't get physically or mentally excited in the evenings. Don't exercise at night. Avoid sex just before bedtime if it leaves you in an excited state. However, some people find sex a release. They may find it easier to sleep right after sex.

- A warm bath may be helpful to induce sleep.

Dr. Peter J. Steincrohn says warm or hot water will raise the body temperature and increase tiredness. Warm water also aids in reducing tension and helps the mind to concentrate on peaceful things, which should make it easier to fall asleep after the bath.

• Progressive relaxation is a simple technique that may also help. Starting with the muscles in your toes, each muscle group is tensed and relaxed several times. By the time you work your way up through your toes, feet, calves, thighs, stomach, and arms, to your neck, you should be very relaxed.

• A glass of warm milk may be helpful. This is an old folk remedy that seems to have scientific basis to help insomnia. Dr. Ernest Hartmann in Boston has shown that L-tryptophan, an amino acid found abundantly in milk, helps people get to sleep easily. According to Dr. Hartmann's research, L-tryptophan stimulates the production of serotonin which is involved in the brain's sleep process. L-tryptophan supplements are available in some health food stores. However, we do not recommend taking these supplements regularly because other research has shown that L-tryptophan supplements may speed the aging process. At this time, it seems that drinking warm milk is the best way to get the benefit of this amino acid. L-tryptophan is also found in other dairy products, as well as in bananas, tuna, sardines (with bones), soybeans and turkey.

• Taking hops, the flower used in flavoring beer, may help lull you to sleep, says Varro E. Tyler, Ph.D., dean of the Schools of Pharmacy, Nursing and Health Sciences at Purdue University. Hops are known for their role in making beer, but they also have a sedative effect, he explains. A few years ago, people who harvested hops were found to become sleepy and tired after just a short time at work in the fields. Their behavior led to the discovery of hops as a sedative, according to Dr. Tyler. For the best sedative effect, Dr. Tyler suggests putting some hops in a muslin or cloth bag and using the bag as a pillow.

• Eat carbohydrates at your evening meal or as the last food you eat before going to bed. Eating meals composed mainly of carbohydrates may help people relax and feel drowsy, according to research at Texas Tech University. Psychology professor Dr. Bonnie Spring measured the difference between the effects of carbohydrate and protein meals in 184 people. Proteins made the people feel tense, but carbohydrates relaxed the men and made the women feel drowsy.

• If insomnia persists after trying the

preceding health tips, try this. Upon awakening at night or experiencing insomnia, get up and stay awake throughout the next day without napping. The next evening your body will be so tired that you will usually have no trouble going to sleep and staying asleep for the entire night. After this, your sleep patterns will be much more regular. If you should experience insomnia again, try the same technique. After you do this several times, your body may adjust to getting just the right amount of sleep each night without awakening.

Easy Way To Get Rid
Of This Sleep Disorder

If you're not getting your quota of sleep because you lie awake in bed for hours every night, here's help.

About two million people with sleep disorders in the U.S. are classified as "sleep onset" insomniacs, according to *Discover* magazine. These people sleep soundly, "but only after hours of tossing and turning."

Researchers at Stanford, Harvard and New York City's Montefiore Hospital found a way to help: resetting an insomniac's biological clock.

Stanford's Charles Czeisler maintains that

sleeping time "coincides with the daily rise and fall of body temperature." When a person's body temperature reaches its low of ninety-seven degrees each day, he becomes sleepy. He awakens as his temperature climbs toward its summit of ninety-nine degrees.

For some reason, the body temperature of sleep-onset insomniacs does not drop until the early morning hours.

Czeisler therefore suggests resetting the insomniac's biological clock by "postponing bedtime a little each night over the course of about a week."

The sleep-onset insomniac should go to bed "several hours later than usual" the first night, and several more hours the next, until nearly an entire day of sleep has been lost. By then the patient should be back to a normal sleeping pattern.

"This process helps readjust the body's metabolic clock, fooling it into dropping body temperature at a decent bedtime," *Discover* concludes.

Natural Ways to Beat Temporary Insomnia

Few things are more frustrating than lying awake in bed knowing you should be sleepy while your body's telling you it's ready to run a marathon.

"Many poor sleepers are more aroused than good sleepers," says sleep specialist Richard R. Bootzin, Ph.D., of Northwestern University. They have higher body temperature and skin resistance, "and more body movements per hour than good sleepers." In other words, their nervous systems are ready for action, not sleep.

We've all experienced temporary insomnia. In the past, doctors have usually prescribed sleeping pills for this frequent disorder. In recent years, though, doctors and psychologists have realized that these drugs either don't work or can be harmful when taken frequently, *Prevention* magazine reports. Researchers are now finding there are simple techniques you can do in your bed that are more effective and less dangerous than drugs.

Muscle relaxation techniques— particularly one called "progressive relaxation"— are one option. Courses in progressive relaxation teach you to identify 16 body muscles and know what tension and relaxation feel like. With practice, people can relax themselves completely in five minutes by consciously relaxing their muscles.

Proper breathing can also help induce sleep. Dr. Beata Jencks advises using your imagination.

Breathe through your finger tips, she says, up the shoulders and then exhale down the trunk and legs and out the toes. To breathe deeply, Dr. Jencks says to imagine your breathing is rising and falling like ocean waves.

"Autogenic training is another natural and potent sleep aid," *Prevention* reports. This is based on the idea that "your mind can compel your body to relax by concentrating on feelings of heaviness and warmth."

An experiment with sixteen college students with insomnia revealed that the time they needed to fall asleep dropped from fifty-two to twenty-two minutes after they focused on warmth and heaviness.

To imagine heaviness, Dr. Jencks suggests you close your eyes, lift one arm a little, and "let it drop heavily," like a Raggedy Ann doll, she says.

Feelings of warmth can be invoked by imagining the same Raggedy Ann Doll being put in the sun, Jencks says. Then imagine you are the doll, and the sun is warming your limbs while your head remains in the shade, nice and cool.

Dr. Quentin Regestein, director of the sleep clinic at Bigham and Women's Hospital in Boston, says pre-bed rituals are important in encouraging sleep. Research has found that people fall asleep more easily when they adhere to a nightly ritual such as brushing their teeth, then "curling into their favorite position," *Prevention* says.

INTELLIGENCE

Nutrients That Help Your Mind

Can a nutritionally poor diet reduce your intelligence level? A study in Wales suggests it can (*Psychology Today*). A psychologist and a school teacher gave 90 Welsh children, ages 12 and 13, verbal and nonverbal intelligence tests. For three days prior to the tests the children kept diaries of what they ate. The children were then split into three groups, one receiving vitamin/mineral supplements, another a pill containing no vitamins or minerals, and a third group no pill at all.

The group that took the supplements "showed a significant increase in nonverbal I.Q. scores," *Psychology Today* reports. The other two groups showed no increase. (Verbal-intelligence test scores were slightly better across the board).

"The findings are consistent with other studies attributing neural function deficits to deficiencies in thiamine, B vitamins, zinc and iron," *Psychology Today* points out. For concerned parents and junk-food junkies, it's further proof that mental states are dependent upon what we eat.

KIDNEY STONES

Shock Waves and Lasers Make Most Kidney Stone Surgery Obsolete

In 1980, Dr. Christian Chaussy of Munich, Germany, used electrically generated shock waves to break up a patient's kidney stone (*Journal of Urology*). No incision was required. In a few days the patient returned to work without so much as a scratch to prove he had been hospitalized.

Known as "extracorporeal shock-wave lithotripsy," or simply "lithotripsy" (ESWL), Dr. Chaussy's treatment has become so popular and successful in America that it may eventually replace surgery as the treatment of choice for kidney stones.

Dr. Stephen P. Dretler, Director of the Lithotriptor unit at Massachusetts General Hospital, explains how ESWL works: A patient is placed in a large tank of water, the kidney stone is located by two x-ray machines, and shock waves of sound are first focused on the stones then transmitted through the water by devices in the tank. The shock waves do not destroy bone or soft tissue, Drettler points out, but break kidney stones because the stones form a unique, "resistance to the passage of sound waves" (*The Harvard Medical School Health Letter*).

The treatment "allows patients to return to normal life almost immediately," Dretler says.

Although x-rays are employed to "image the stones," tests reveal that the amount of radiation compares "favorably with exposure rates...for other routine radiological procedures," according to the *Journal of Urology*. The amount of radiation received depends on the size and location of the stone and the number of shocks required.

Lithotripsy technology has advanced rapidly. New machines can now disintegrate stones on an outpatient basis, according to the *Medical Tribune*.

The Lithostar machine, currently being tested at four U.S. medical centers, is much less costly than the older model bathtub ESWL.

The machine is held directly against the body and sends a mild shock wave through a steel membrane. Because the Lithostar requires only a local anesthetic, the procedure can be done on an outpatient basis. If a small stone is being treated, a patient may return to work the next day.

Dr. Bruce McClennan has used the Lithostar on more than 225 patients and says it reportedly feels "like getting hit with a fly swatter." "Afterwards there's no nausea, no vomiting," McClennan adds.

Another new machine, the Candela Laser Lithotripter, has already been approved by the FDA. Intended to treat only those patients unable to undergo traditional ESWL, the *Medical Tribune* says, it has become a popular alternative because of its low cost.

Hospitals usually charge about $250- $500 for a Candela machine treatment, compared with $3,500 for the other machines.

The Candela laser is less likely to damage surrounding tissue than shock wave treatments. General anesthesia may be required but a patient should still be back to work in two to three days, compared with six weeks required after surgical stone removal, the *Medical Tribune* reports.

LEAD POISONING

Danger From Your Fireplace

Burning newspapers in woodstoves or private fireplaces can increase the lead content in the home to dangerous levels, warns the *New England Journal of Medicine* (297:17,943).

Small amounts of newspaper can be used to start a fire, but logs of rolled newspapers or newspapers with colored ink should *not be burned* because they'll add too much lead to the air. The lead content in newspapers comes from the ink.

Lead poisoning can damage the brain, bones, kidneys, liver, and central nervous system and has been linked to cancer (*Journal of the American Medical Association* 237:24,2627) so high concentrations of lead should be avoided (*The New England Journal of Medicine* 316:17,1037). Initial signs of lead poisoning include abdominal pain, loss of appetite, nausea, vomiting, unusual illnesses, headaches, irritability and anemia.

Poisoned By
A Dietary Supplement?

Calcium supplements containing bone meal often contain lead, and large doses of the bone meal could cause lead poisoning, scientists from the University of Illinois warn.

Many women use large daily doses of bone meal as a calcium supplement, since it is cheaper than most other sources of calcium. However, bone meal is not technically a drug or food, so the labeling and quality control for it is not as stringent as it is for regular calcium supplements.

LONGEVITY

Why Cynics Die Young

Which of these statements do you agree with: (1) "People are basically honest," or (2) "In a time of crises, people will generally look out for themselves." Your response may reveal as much about your longevity as your opinion of human nature.

Researchers at Duke University have found that "a suspicious or mistrustful frame of mind can be a significant factor in premature death," according to *Discover* magazine.

Begun in 1969, the study started with 500 men and women filling out personality surveys "designed to measure suspiciousness or the tendency to have negative thoughts about the motives of other people," *Discover* reports. Questions were similar to the above examples, and those who took the survey were ranked low to high on a 100-point suspiciousness scale.

After 15 years, 145 of the 500 people had died. The researchers examined causes of death and analyzed the data. The found "a significantly higher percentage of people with low suspiciousness scores were still alive," psychiatrist

Redford Williams, Jr., of Duke University Medical Center says. People whose suspiciousness scale was in the eighties had a 40 percent greater chance of dying than those in the twentieth percentile, Williams adds. Even more disturbing is that the suspiciousness evidenced was not abnormal. "It's very common behavior," he says. "It's simply that it happens to be not very good for you."

The obvious question is: How can suspiciousness be harmful to your health? Duke psychologist John Barfoot says the key is not suspiciousness itself "but the way that suspicious people live their lives." Barfoot speculates that people who are not suspicious have better social relationships that act as a buffer against everyday irritants. Cynical or mistrustful people may have an equal number of relationships, but they're less satisfying, he says. Suspicious people, therefore, have "less opportunity for relying on others to help cope with stress, and that can mean greater likelihood of stress-related death," he concludes.

Why Do Women Live Longer Than Men?

Women live longer than men—in industrialized nations four to ten years longer, according to *The Health Letter*. Why?

Men begin having heart attacks in their thirties and the rate increases through their forties and fifties. Women, however, don't usually have heart attacks until after menopause. By age 65 the death rate from heart attacks in women and men is about equal. This is attributed primarily to hormone differences.

Testosterone causes men to have lower levels of the "good" HDL cholesterol and more of the "bad" cholesterol LDL, *The Health Letter* reports. Estrogen appears to have just the opposite effect.

There is even a theory that women have an inherited gene that contributes to longevity. Women have xx chromosomes, men have xy chromosomes. It is thought that two x chromosomes may allow the female to "select the best gene on either x chromosome." The male can only use the one gene that happens to be on his x chromosome, according to the theory.

A study of an Amish family in which the men had a chromosomal abnormality seems to support this theory. The men in that family lived an average of 82.3 years, the women only 77.4 years. Who is the weaker sex after all?

NAIL PROBLEMS

Brittle Nails? This Nutrient Can Make Them Strong

Brittle nails indicate a nutrient deficiency, according to *Prevention* magazine. Researchers in Sheffield, England, discovered that a "shortage of iron in the nail seems to be a sign of iron-deficiency anemia."

The research found that five women who suffered from iron-deficiency anemia also had brittle nails. After supplements with iron, however, the nails weren't brittle anymore.

The link between iron and brittle nails is an example of how nail condition may signal the presence of more serious health problems.

"Certain changes in the nails' appearance and chemical content may be warning flags that pop up years in advance of actual disease," *Prevention* says. Researchers are beginning to see nails as "a major diagnostic tool of the future...a window on the inner processes of the body." So if you notice changes in the texture or color of your nails it would be wise to see a doctor.

OSTEOPOROSIS

Easy Exercise Prevents Bone Loss

A recent study at the University of Oregon conducted with postmenopausal women suggests that a moderate exercise program may reduce bone deterioration in the elderly.

According to an article in *Prevention* magazine, the study involved twelve active and twelve sedentary elderly women. The participants who exercised a minimum of fifty minutes, three times a week, experienced biochemical changes which increased bone density. The exercises used in the study, such as lifting the chest and head off the floor, strengthened and contracted muscles in the back.

As reported in *Health Confidential,* osteoporosis is a weakening of bone matter that leads to brittle bones and bent-over posture suffered by twenty-four million Americans. This figure includes fifty percent of women over age forty-five and ninety percent of women over seventy-five.

If you fall into this category, make sure you consult your physician before beginning any exercise program to improve your health.

Stretch Your Bones Into Shape

Doctors are discovering you can strengthen your spine through back extension exercises.

Doctors at the Mayo Clinic found that the stronger the back-straightening muscles were, the greater the bone mineral density of the spinal bones, according to *Prevention* magazine .

They measured the bone mineral density of the spine and the strength of the back extensor muscles (the ones used when the back is arched) of 68 healthy postmenopausal women to reach their conclusion.

Exercise has been linked to bone density before, but this study is the first to find a "specific correlation between the vertebrae and their closely related muscles," *Prevention* says.

One of the Mayo Clinic doctors, Mehrsheed Sinaki, notes that the muscles, "directly attached to the bones play the biggest role." He suggests doing extension exercises such as "arching and straightening the back."

"Women with osteoporosis who did these exercises had less than one-third the spinal fractures than those doing bending exercises or no exercise," the article reports.

Doctors even wonder now if loss of calcium

from the vertebrae can be halted or reversed by strengthening back muscles.

Risk of Hip Fracture Reduced by Hormone Treatment

As we grow older our bones become progressively brittle and break easier. For a large segment of the population that risk can now be reduced.

Findings of the Framingham study, going on since 1948, offer a ray of hope to postmenopausal women, the *Harvard Medical School Health Letter,* reports. The study monitored almost 3,000 women and found that estrogen taken almost any time after menopause cuts the risk of hip fracture by a third. Those who took estrogen for two years reduced their risks by two-thirds.

Although it has not been determined what the ideal duration and dose of estrogen should be, the evidence that estrogen protects against broken bones is almost conclusive.

There is speculation that taking estrogen after menopause increases the risk of endometrial cancer. However taking the hormone progestin with the estrogen reduces that risk. The *Harvard Medical School Health Letter* also emphasizes that endometrial cancer develops slowly and is easily detected by endometrial biopsy at an early stage.

Restore Bones Damaged By Osteoporosis

Is it possible to reverse the effects of the bone-thinning disease osteoporosis? That's what doctors are saying of the drug didronel.

"It's a fantastic, inexpensive drug that appears to be better than anything else we have today for the treatment of osteoporosis," says Dr. Paul Miller, of the University of Colorado's Health Science Center.

Osteoporosis saps calcium from the bones, causing fractures in millions of people each year, particularly postmenopausal women.

Of 50 women with osteoporosis who took didronel as part of a study at the University of Colorado, 70 percent "have shown significant gains in bone mass," Miller reports. "That means their bones are actually becoming thicker and stronger as they take the drug, decreasing their risk of fractures."

Miller states that some of the women experienced a 39 percent increase in bone mass and the average increase was 17 percent.

The 70 percent success rate of the University of

Colorado study has been duplicated in other studies in the U.S., France and Denmark.

"The most important result of didronel treatment is that the gain in bone mass seems to be maintained for at least three years," says Dr. Ole Sorensen of Sunby Hospital in Copenhagen, Denmark.

While didronel appears to have no major side effects, "it may cause some gastrointestinal discomfort and can also trigger a mild skin rash," Dr. Frederic McDuffie, Medical Director of the Arthritis Foundation, says.

Didronel has been approved by the U.S. Food and Drug Administration but, as yet, only for the bone disorder Pagets' disease, Dr. Miller says.

If a doctor feels the drug may be helpful for an osteoporosis sufferer, however, he can prescribe it, Miller says.

Build Stronger Bones By Swimming

Swimming is known to be excellent for the cardiovascular system. But for the bones?

Prevention magazine cites results of a study done at the Veterans Administration Medical Center in Portland, Oregon, suggesting such a link. A group of older men who had been swimming many years was compared with a group of sedentary men of similar age. The swimmers swam an average of 4.6 hours a week for thirteen years.

The vertebrae of the swimmers was found to be "12 percent denser than those of the nonswimmers," *Prevention* reports.

It had previously been thought that only so-called weight-bearing activities like walking or running maintained strong bones. Dr. Eric S. Orwell, the chief researcher of the study, says that weight bearing on the bones may not be as crucial for increased bone mass as force exerted on the bones by the muscles. He adds: "You can exert a tremendous amount of force on the skeleton by the muscular action of swimming."

Swimming is also helpful for those with arthritis, osteoporosis or other bone and joint disorders.

Antacids That Affect Your Bones

You were probably thinking of your stomach and not your bones when you took that antacid. However, antacids have ingredients that can make a big difference to the health of your bones.

Avoid antacids that contain aluminum. Aluminum draws phosphorus out of the bones and makes the body more susceptible to osteoporosis. Antacids containing aluminum include: Camalox®, Delcid®, Di-Gel®, Gaviscon®, Gelusil-M®, Gelusil-II®, Maalox®, Maalox Plus®, Nephrox®, Tempo®, WinGel®, ALternaGEL®, Aludrox®, Amphojel®, Mylanta®, Mylanta-II®, and Simeco®. Large amounts of these taken over long periods of time may be very harmful to your bones.

Antacids like Tums®, which have only calcium carbonate as an active ingredient, actually have a protective effect — they provide calcium necessary for healthy bones and prevention of osteoporosis. Although Tums® and some other antacids contain calcium, some doctors do not recommend using antacids for a daily calcium supplement because in large quantities they may aggravate your digestive system and cause constipation.

Be Careful When Taking This Drug

If you are taking prednisone (Deltasone®) or other corticosteroids you are at increased risk of developing osteoporosis, reports a Canadian doctor.

Dr. Jonathon Adachi of St. Joseph's Hospital in Hamilton, Ontario, says that men and women who are taking this drug should probably take extra vitamins D and Calcium because of this added risk.

Since osteoporosis develops over a long period of time, using proper precautions now are important.

PAIN

Ten Easy Ways to Avoid Pain

If you have suffered from chronic pain in your neck, you know what a "pain in the neck" it can be to get rid of. But relief might be easier than you think.

According to Dr. Ron Lawrence, a neurologist at UCLA, over half of the chronic neck and back pain, tension headaches and even foot discomforts suffered by millions of people can be relieved by following these simple hints, reports *The National Enquirer*.

• *Wear a comfortable shoe.* It shouldn't be too big or too small. The proper shoe will support your arch, prevent development of corns and calliusses, and absorb the shock each step places on your feet.

• *Don't run or walk on hard surfaces.* Not only can veins and leg muscles suffer, joints in the hips and knees can be damaged. For exercise, try walking on grass or dirt trails if possible. If your only choice is concrete floors or outside pavement, try other methods of aerobic exercise. If you stand for long periods of time, try adding carpeting or a mat to make the surface softer. Many cashiers or people who stand at work find that one or two mats will help buffer the effects of a concrete floor.

- *Lift objects properly, regardless of weight.* A lot of back pain is caused by improper use of the back muscles when lifting even light objects. Improper lifting can also place stress on the joints. Always bend your knees, squat down, bend your elbows and then lift with you whole body. Never straighten your legs completely, or twist your spine from side to side while lifting an object.

- *Sleep face up—never down.* Poor sleeping habits can lead to stiff joints and sore muscles. If you've ever had a "catch" in the neck or shoulder, you know how painful this can be. Make sure you have adequate head, foot and side room for sleeping. If you must sleep on your abdomen, place a pillow under your stomach or bend one or both knees to the side for added support.

- *Watch where and how you sit.* Office and auto seats, for example, may place excess stress on the lower back. Some types of seats support the mid-back, but not the lower back. Always sit so that your natural spinal curve is not in any stress. Sit erect and when possible elevate your feet slightly.

- *Watch your body position.* Reading in bed, watching television, sudden head movements and even holding a phone between your neck and shoulder can result in neck pain and headaches. Never read in bed with your head propped up by a pillow. Instead, sit erect and place a pillow under your knees for back support. When watching TV, make sure the set is at eye level or slightly above. Don't hold the phone between your head and shoulder, but keep your head straight and hold the phone to the ear with your hand. If you must use a telephone for long periods of time, buy an inexpensive headset to keep your head erect and your hands free. Always move your head slowly and in one motion. Never jerk your head quickly into any position.

• *Take care of your hands*. Improper hand care can lead to pain from the elbow to the fingertips. Keep you hands flexible by massaging them two or three minute daily. Squeezing a soft rubber ball can promote strength and flexibility in hand muscles. Wear gloves while doing yard work or other jobs that place stress on hands and that may result in cuts and scratches.

• *Use a good source of light*. Eye stress is a major cause of occasional headaches. To prevent eyestrain, use 60 watt bulbs for lamps and light fixtures. Always read with the light coming over the shoulder, not directly in the eyes. This is especially important for demanding visual tasks like reading, watching TV, cooking and handicrafts.

• *Don't overeat.* Overeating stresses the stomach muscles and creates a potbelly. This in turn can lead to back and neck pain. If you can't control your appetite, try drinking a glass of water or eating a small salad before your meal.

• *Exercise.* Most chronic pain is caused by lack of exercise. If the muscles are not in shape they cannot support the joints properly and a "chain reaction" of pain is started. Try some form of exercise daily. Walking is a great choice. When possible walk to your destination, instead of riding in your car.

When Remedies Do More Harm Than Good

Got a headache? Maybe a cup of coffee and a couple aspirin will help.

Not necessarily, according to Dr. Alan Rapoport, director of the New England Center for Headache. Overuse of painkillers can cause a lack of effectiveness in most people and some people even suffer "rebound" headaches actually caused by the drugs, says Rapoport.

Overuse of painkillers lowers the body's own natural pain killing ability, Dr. Rapoport explains.

People taking up to six tablets of daily acetaminophen (Tylenol®) or aspirin products can be affected and should try gradual withdrawal. He suggests discussing biofeedback or other pain-killing alternatives with your doctor.

And as for the coffee—caffeine dependence can make you more sensitive to pain, says Dr. Norma Shealy, Director of the Shealy Institute for Comprehensive Pain and Health Care in Missouri. Since caffeine acts as a stimulant and activates adrenaline, Dr. Shealy recommends completely eliminating caffeine to help reduce chronic pain.

On the other hand, when you really do need a pain pill, those that contain both aspirin and caffeine are reported to be more effective than just plain aspirin.

A Flavoring That Can Cause Severe Pain

Don't eat bay leaves! Bay leaves are used for flavoring in many tomato-based foods like spaghetti, but they should be removed before the food is served. Recently a man was admitted into an emergency room with "the worst pain he had ever experienced." The stem of a bay leaf was discovered in his anal passage. Bay leaves that have been eaten can cause severe pain and damage to many internal organs, yet they are often overlooked during an emergency. Please remember to remove bay leaves from your food and never chew or swallow one.

Does Chiropractic Treatment Help?

Many people with backaches or other aches and pains pay frequent visits to chiropractors. Chiropractic treatment can hardly be called a natural way of dealing with physical problems, because it involves taking x-rays and manipulating the spine by a skilled practitioner. Some medical doctors claim that there is no value to chiropractic treatment and that most chiropractors are quacks. S. me chiropractors respond that medical doctors don't care about the total well-being of their patients and often deal with them in a detached, impersonal manner.

A wise medical doctor once was asked what he thought of chiropractic treatment, and he said that at least one-half of what physicians and other healers do is give the patient assurance that he's going to get better because of a particular type of treatment. Later, the patient often will get better, regardless of whether the treatment itself helped him.

This "placebo" effect is responsible for much of

the healing that takes place regardless of what sort of treatment is used or what sort of practitioner used the treatment. According to the medical doctor, most chiropractors excel in the area of giving the patient confidence that he will get better because of their treatment.

When the "placebo" effect is combined with the body's own God-given ability to heal itself, the work of chiropractors, if they are sincerely interested in the welfare of their patients and if they are careful not to injure the spine, may sometimes surpass that of standard medical treatment.

Is there any benefit to chiropractic treatment in addition to the helpful psychological aspects? One scientific study which attempted to answer this question showed that patients who were treated for lower back pain through typical chiropractic manipulations experience more relief from pain than other patients who were treated in a different way as a control population. Unfortunately, this study showed the total healing time of the patients treated with chiropractic manipulation was greater than the patients in the control group.

There are not many good scientific studies on the effectiveness of chiropractic treatment. On the positive side, it seems to make some people feel better, and many people testify to this. On the negative side, many medical doctors point out that it is quite possible to seriously injure the spine by manipulation and to cause injury to other parts of the body. One recent study by an M.D. showed that many elderly people experienced strokes soon after receiving chiropractic manipulation in the neck area. Medical doctors caution that spinal manipulation is less dangerous when it is performed in the lower back than when it is performed in the neck or upper back.

A Simple Device That May Help

Do you ever which you could push a button and get rid of some of that pain? Now there is a device that may help.

A portable box which can be worn on your hip delivers mild electrical stimulation to the area of chronic pain. This reduces pain in most people, because the current activates the body's nerves The box is like a paging device, and you can control the amount of stimulation you'll receive. Known as TENS (transcutaneous electrical nerve stimulation), many pain clinics are using these simple devices to help people cope with chronic and sudden pain.

POISON IVY

A New Wonder Drug?

The itching and swelling of poison ivy may soon be a thing of the past, thanks to a new vaccine especially for this irritating infection.

Dr. William Epstein at the University of California in San Francisco explains that the vaccine has proven effective in animals, but more tests are needed before the poison ivy vaccine will be approved for the general public.

PREGNANCY

How Keeping This Pet
May HarmYour Unborn Baby

Your cat looks so peaceful and innocent lying there beside you, but did you know it can carry a parasite that is potentially hazardous for your unborn child?

A parasitic infection called toxoplasmosis can be transmitted by contaminated cat feces and may seriously injure the unborn child. Toxoplasmosis is highly contagious. In adults the toxoplasmosis may cause a minor illness much like the flu. However, for an unborn baby, toxoplasmosis in the mother can be extremely dangerous. During pregnancy the litter box should be emptied and cleaned daily, but not by the pregnant mother, the Public Health Service recommends

Usually it is safe for a pregnant mother to keep a cat in her hom during her pregnancy if a veterinarian has examined the cat to prove it doesn't have the infection. The mother-to-be should not have any contact with cat urine or feces, and she should wash her hands thoroughly after touching the cat.

A Simple Way To Help Prevent Stillbirths

To reduce the possibility of stillbirths, women in the seventh to ninth months of pregnancy just need to count how often their babies kick. Dr. Kathleen Piacquadio of San Diego reported the results of a study involving over 1,500 women to the American College of Obstetricians and Gynecologists. Piacquadio found that counting the kicks during this critical trimester of pregnancy dropped the rate of fetal deaths from 8.7 to 2.1 deaths per 1,000.

The women were instructed to count how many times each day their babies kicked within a specific two-hour period. They were told to note the number of kicks for two hours in the evening, preferably between 7 and 10 p.m. when the baby is most active. If the count was less than ten kicks, the women were to go directly to a hospital because of the possibility that the umbilical cord was caught around the baby's neck.

Most times, a low count will not be serious, but only further tests by a doctor can insure the baby's health. In serious cases, an emergency Cesarean Section can be performed and the baby's life saved, Piacquadio says.

Don't Use This Product To Cut Back on Calories During Pregnancy

Watching your calories during pregnancy is commendable, but be careful that you don't injure your baby in the process.

A new study shows that high amounts of NutraSweet® can cause birth defects. NutraSweet® increases the level of phenylalanine, an amino acid known to cause birth defects in certain enzyme deficient babies with PKU. Dr. Reuben Matalon at the University of Illinois recommends that pregnant women cut out NutraSweet® or limit their intake to a maximum of three diet soft drinks per day.

NutraSweet® is the ingredient found in Equal® and many types of low-calorie products, including most diet soft drinks.

PRESCRIPTION DRUGS

A New Way To Take
Your Medicine

Follow your doctor's and pharmacist's advice about your prescriptions. The Ninth Schering Report estimates that "125,000 Americans die each year simply because they fail to take their medicine as prescribed. That's the worst case, but almost equally distressful is the unnecessary extra hundreds of thousands of hospitalizations." The Schering Report also noted that about one-third of patients don't have their prescriptions refilled as the doctor ordered. Since many medications are only effective on a long-term basis, people are short-changing their health when they try to "play doctor" with their prescriptions. Forgetful patients may get help soon, though.

There's a new way to take your medicine: no shots and no pills. Small patches that are applied to your skin like a band-aid are revolutionizing medicine. The patches, known as transdermal patches since the medicine enters the body through the skin, are now being used for many different types of medicine. Three brands of nitroglycerin patches are already available. The skin patches allow the drugs to be released directly into the system and provides a more constant level of medicine than a pill that is swallowed. The oral drug would be released in one large dose, but the skin patch provides an even level of medication over a longer time period. The lower dose and longer time of delivery also help reduce some side drug side effects. Many patches have to be replaced only once a week, so they are easier to remember and more convenient than pills.

How to Get Medicine
Free for the Asking

Have you ever gotten a big surprise when you've taken a prescription for a new drug to your pharmacist and then found out how much it costs? "Sixty dollars please," isn't uncommon to hear at the cash register these days. However, you may be able to get your medicine at no charge.

Doctors are flooded with free samples of drugs from pharmaceutical companies, especially samples of the newest and most expensive drugs. Ask your doctor if he has any samples of a drug he has prescribed for you. You'll be surprised at how often he says yes, especially if you're in financial need. He may have just your drug or a good alternative on hand, but he probably won't think to volunteer this information. So be sure to ask, and maybe you'll get a pleasant surprise.

PROSTATE

Prostate Surgery Might Be A Thing
Of The Past

Prostate surgery is common among middle-aged men. The biggest reason: a non-cancerous tumor called "benign prostatic hyperplasia (BPH)."

Dr. Patrick C. Walsh calls BPH an "almost universal phenomenon" and cites studies which suggest that it affects 80 percent of men 40 or older, according to the *Medical Tribune* .

Until now, the only effective therapy was surgery, but treatment being perfected at the University of Southern California (USC) might change that. The technique is transurethral hyperthermia, an adaption of a transrectal procedure developed in Israel.

The Israeli technique, which involves heating the prostate, has prompted a physicist at USC to equip a catheter with microwave antennas and temperature-sensing systems. The catheter can be "introduced through the penis and the urethra and anchored in the bladder with a balloon," *Medical Tribune* says.

The catheter then heats the central portion of the gland from which the obstructive symptoms eminate.

The article says the procedure "appears to shrink tumor tissue, thus relieving pressure on the urethra and causing symptoms to diminish or disappear."

The Israeli doctors have reported an 80 percent success rate, and the researchers at USC hope to improve on that score.

Dr. Michael D. Sapozink of USC states: "The ultimate goal, of course, is to be able to provide a nonsurgical form of treatment for a very common disease that distresses a lot of men."

Good News For Patients Facing Prostate Surgery

A new prostate procedure saves sexual function. In the past, men facing prostate surgery also faced the strong possibility of impotency. Now, there's hope.

Dr. Patrick Walsh at Johns Hopkins University has identified the microscopic nerves that control an erection. With skillful surgery, the nerves can be avoided and full potency can be kept.

The nerves were difficult to identify because they are contained in a bundle with blood vessels, Walsh reports. Now surgeons can make an incision closer to the prostate. The new location of the incision also causes less loss of bladder or bowel control.

Prostate surgery that avoids these nerves has been successfully completed in over five hundred men in New York and Boston and is becoming widely used throughout the U.S., Walsh explains.

PSORIASIS

A Nutrient That May Clear Up Your Skin

Dr. Michael F. Holick, the director of the Vitamin D, Skin and Bone Research Laboratory at Boston City Hospital, is excited about his latest research on psoriasis.

His researchers have found that an "active form of vitamin D is able to inhibit the growth of skin cells" which cause psoriasis, he says.

Until now, no treatment for the scaly, itchy skin of psoriasis has been completely effective or free of side effects, *Prevention* magazine reports.

The results of Dr. Holick's research, recently published in the *Archives of Dermatology*, offer the most promising news for psoriasis sufferers yet.

"Sixty percent of our patients respond to this therapy," Holick says. Redness and scales on the scalp have decreased markedly, and their lesions eventually cleared up.

Further research of two hundred psoriasis patients will be conducted this year to make sure there are no side effects to the drug.

Holick notes that store-bought vitamin D will be "of no use for treating psoriasis," and that taken in large doses it can be toxic. For right now, the psoriasis-fighting form of vitamin D is available only in Holick's study.

For psoriasis sufferers, approval of the new drug will be a welcome relief.

Vitamins to Help Your Skin?

Derivatives of vitamin A are used as prescription treatments for acne, so although vitamin A is not routinely given for psoriasis, it is known to help the skin. Vitamin A maintains the smoothness, health and functioning of the skin and the mucous membranes. Vitamin A also helps build body protein and promotes the growth of body tissues.

However, large doses of vitamin A can cause severe side effects so doctors warn against taking more than the RDA (Recommended Dietary Allowance) — 5,000 International Units (I.U.'s) daily for adult males and 4,000 I.U.'s for adult females. Vitamin A can be obtained naturally by eating healthy amounts of fruits and vegetables, particularly yellow vegetables like carrots or squash, liver or taking cod liver oil.

You can also get vitamin A by eating liver or taking cod liver oil.

One Couple's Story

Here's an interesting story we received from a reader. If you want to try her remedy, check with your doctor. Large doses of vitamin A or D, especially if taken over a long period of time, can cause serious side effects.

Since our marriage in 1952, and back into his teenage years, my husband Red was plagued with psoriasis. Some years after our marriage he mentioned to me, "I am so glad summer is coming. My psoriasis goes away when I get out in the sun."

Something plagued me about that statement, until I remembered from grade school days that "vitamins A and D are the sunshine vitamins." (Editor's Note: Only Vitamin D is "the sunshine vitamin .) *Red was not a pill-taker, but he was so miserable with psoriasis on his arms from above the elbow to the wrist and covering most of his lower abdomen, back and front of his body, I bought him a bottle of chewable A and D vitamins. (Red did not like to swallow pills at that point in his life.)*

Every day I reminded him to take a couple. From that day forward, all he had to do was take those vitamins during the times when the miserable itching skin condition began to return.

The point is, when he took the A and D vitamins his psoriasis slowly disappeared — not too slowly, at that. During the later years, for the last 20 years, he had no psoriasis at all. The minute it began to appear, he knew exactly what to do.

—Mrs. L.K.N., Abington, PA.

RECTAL ITCHING

Foods to Avoid to Get Relief

Coffee and dairy products cause over 90 percent of rectal itching problems, reports Dr. William Friend at the University of Washington. Large amounts of vitamin C, tomatoes, tea, cola drinks, chocolate, and beer are also known to cause itching in the rectum. To stop the problem, Dr. Friend suggests using a hydrocortisone cream and eliminating the offending foods from your diet.

Rectal itching can be caused by mites and other problems. Be sure to check with your doctor.

SCOLIOSIS

Spinal Curve Straightened Without Surgery

Many of us live with minor skeletal abnormalities that never bother us: a leg one-fourth inch shorter than the other or a slightly stooped shoulder, for instance.

As much as two percent of the population have small curves (10 to 20 degrees), in their back, says *The Western Journal of Medicine*. Such a minor curve may cause a shoulder to stoop but otherwise should be of no concern. When the curve progresses beyond 20 degrees, however, a person may have scoliosis.

Defined as a "lateral curvature of the spine," scoliosis is most common in adolescents, particularly girls. If severe enough, surgery may be required.

Until recently the most common treatment for scoliosis was the wearing of a brace. Bulky and noticeable, a brace is worn up to 23 hours a day for one to five years. To an adolescent, a brace is often as psychologically difficult as it is physically uncomfortable. Also, after brace removal the spine gradually reverts to its previous curvature.

Now there is another non-surgical treatment for

scoliosis. It uses electricity to stimulate the muscles surrounding the spinal curve. Called "lateral electrical percutaneous muscle stimulation," the treatment has been effective in halting progression of a spinal curve in eighty-five percent of the cases, reports *The Western Journal of Medicine*. The electrical stimulation comes from "electrode leads," wired to a battery-powered pulse generator. It is used only eight to twelve hours a day during sleep.

Despite the initial success, doctors see uncertainties. Some doctors have reported success with curves greater than thirty degrees. Others say that for curves over thirty-five degrees, electrical stimulation could not arrest the progress of the curve and surgery was required, according to the article.

The new treatment is popular with patients. The *Journal* notes that problems with depression and low self-esteem that often accompany the brace don't exist where the new treatment is employed.

SENILITY

Senile? It May Only Be A Nutrient You're Missing

Senile dementia, which manifests itself in mental failure, is thought to be genetically based, according to *Lancet*. That prognosis does not leave those afflicted with it much hope.

To deal with a genetically-based disorder requires some medical way of modifying or blocking a chemical process, *Lancet* reports.

Based on research and examination of other genetically-based diseases, Burnet believes the root of dementia may be a simple lack of an important nutrient: zinc. Burnet cites the congenital childhood disease acrodermatitis enteropathica as an example of zinc effectiveness on genetically-based disorders. Zinc supplements remove the accompanying symptoms of skin rash and diarrhea. Since infants with acrodermatitis enteropathica often take in enough zinc in their diets, Burnet speculates the disease is caused by "some genetic anomaly in the absorption or utilization of the available zinc." It is reasonable to suggest, he adds, that genetic-based zinc deficiency may be relatively common.

Dementia basically involves a loss of neurons (nerve cells), Burnet says. He believes neurons die because of some genetic error within them, which, because of age, causes loss of ability to make zinc available.

While cell death is normal as we age, the "devastating fallout of neurons in dementia," Burnet thinks, is due to lack of zinc.

Although more research should be done to confirm his idea, Burnet believes zinc supplements might be the answer for many dementia patients. The recommended daily dietary allowance of zinc for adults is 15 mg. per day.

Burnet's opinion is reinforced by a British doctor, Roy Hullin, who found lower levels of zinc in people who were senile than in people who were not senile. Dr. Hullin feels that the elderly do not get enough zinc in their diets. Zinc is plentiful in meats and seafood.

It's Not Always What You Think

If an older person seems disoriented or confused, don't assume too quickly that he is becoming senile.

A severe drop in body temperature can mimic the signs of senility, warns Dr. Robert Pozos from the University of Minnesota. Confusion, dis-orientation, loss of memory and slurred speech can be caused by a drop in body temperature. Since many older people are less sensitive to cold, they may allow their body temperatures to drop below 97.0° and be misdiagnosed as "senile." People with low body temperatures should be wrapped in warm clothing and blankets and given warm liquids to drink. If the symptoms of senility still exist, the person should be taken to a doctor, Dr. Pozos suggests.

As many as 2.5 million older Americans are especially vulnerable to cold sensitivity, the National Institute on Aging reports. The people are highest risk are: those who are sick or frail, those who are very old, those who live alone, those who are poor and can't afford adequate heat, those who don't shiver, those with kidney problems, overactive thyroid or hypoglycemia, those who drink a lot of alcohol and those on prescription drugs.

Is Your Forgetfulness A Symptom?

"I must be getting old," you find yourself saying when you've forgotten someone's name you thought you'd remember.

But forgetting names is not necessarily a sign of

senility, according to the *Textbook of Medicine* by Beeson and McDermott. People of all ages forget names at times, but as we become older we seem to be more sensitive of our forgetfulness. Losing our ability to grasp *ideas* is a sign of senility, reports the textbook, but occasionally forgetting *names* is quite normal.

Here's a helpful hint to learn and remember someone's name. It seems that many people fail to remember a new person's name because they are really not paying attention during the introduction. Most people are so anxious to introduce themselves, that they miss the new name. Try repeating the new person's name as you introduce yourself, to make sure that you've heard and remembered his name. For example, say "Hi, George. My name is . . ." Try it. You'll be amazed at how simple it is once you learn to listen for the new name and repeat it.

Supplements To Counteract Senility

Senility is memory loss, disorientation, confusion and loss of reasoning ability with advancing age. There is a difference between the natural slowing of our reaction time with advancing age and being senile. Only a small percentage of older Americans suffer from true senility.

Good nutrition and other practices that promote good health may help prevent senility.

Pantothenic acid (vitamin B5) supplements may improve symptoms of senility and depression when taken with other B vitamins.

SHYNESS

A Prescription Drug Can Help

"Shyness," according to the American Heritage Dictionary, "implies either a retiring or withdrawn nature or timidity resulting from lack of social experience."

However, there is a new study that reports that shyness can also be caused by a chemical imbalance in the brain, and it may be possible to treat it with prescription drugs already in use.

Brain fluid removed from the spines of outgoing and shy people revealed low levels of dopamine in the shy people. Dopamine is a chemical found in the brain that helps transmit nerve impulses. Antidepressant drugs, known as monoamine oxidase (MAO) inhibitors, help increase or maintain high dopamine levels and may be used to fight shyness in the future.

SKIN PROBLEMS

Look Better Naturally

Taking care of your skin can help you look better and also avoid other health problems. Here are some tips for improving your complexion:

• Rub your hands together briskly before applying make-up, moisturizer, cleanser or fresheners to the face. Vera Brown, a skin care specialist on the TV program *Hour Magazine*, says that this provides warmth to the face and helps improve the circulation. When cleansing the skin, you should use a warm facecloth, according to Ms. Brown. As well as increasing circulation, the warmth will help open the pores.

Always be gentle when cleansing or touching the membranes under the eyes, the skin specialist warns. These membranes are very tender and can be easily damaged.

• As you get older you should wear less make-up, Vera Brown says. Since make-up accents wrinkles, she believes less make-up is more flattering to an older woman.

• For a good-looking complexion, she recommends a healthful diet. Eliminate coffee, sugar, salt, fried foods and dairy products for the best possible skin appearance.

• Smoking increases wrinkles, according to a study published in the *British Medical Journal.* Wrinkles around the eyes and lips, odd colored complexions, dry skin and leathery skin are more likely to occur in heavy smokers, the study reports.

• Dr. James Fulton believes that acne and skin problems may be provoked by vitamin supplements and foods that contain iodine. Dr. Fulton works at the Acne Research Institute in Newport Beach, California.

• Psoriasis, acne and poor skin color and appearance are often caused by a diet that is low in the mineral zinc. Zinc is found naturally in liver, seafood, dairy products, meat, eggs and whole-grain products.

• You should protect your skin from overexposure to the sun's ultraviolet rays to guard against skin cancer and wrinkles.

New research at Cornell University shows that ultraviolet rays actually destroy beta-carotene. Beta-carotene is a natural substance used by the body to create Vitamin A. Vitamin A has anti-cancer properties which help prevent lung cancer, bladder cancer and skin cancer. To protect yourself agains ultraviolet rays, use a sunscreen with a SPF (sun protection factor) of at least 15 and avoid unnecessary exposure to sunlight.

However, as you protect your skin from the sun's harmful rays, recognize that you may not be getting enough vitamin D. A study in the *Journal of Clinical Investigation* showed that older skin does not produce as much vitamin D from the sun as younger skin does. Vitamin D is important for healthy teeth and bones, for muscle tone, and for kidney function. Many other vitamins and minerals also need vitamin D to work properly. The sun is the best source of vitamin D, although fish, liver, eggs and fortified milk are also good sources. Eat one of these foods each day to get enough vitamin D. Vitamin D supplements that don't exceed the RDA may also be recommended for people who stay out of the sun.

• Common skin tags may be a warning signal of colon cancer. Skin tags are small flaps of skin, usually occurring in groups in the neck, armpit and groin areas. Researchers at the Mount Sinai School of Medicine in New York have discovered that 86 percent of their patients with colon polyps, which often become cancerous, also had skin tags. In further testing, 69 percent of their patients with skin tags also had colon polyps. Until now, skin tags were thought to be harmless but cosmetically annoying. If skin tags are annoying, your doctor can remove them. However, the researchers at

Mount Sinai suggest that, to be safe, anyone with skin tags should have their stools checked for blood. Since a test for occult (hidden) blood in the stool is a simple and inexpensive procedure, it would be well to be safe and have the test.

• Age spots, the little brown blemishes that often appear later in life, may be helped by pantothenic acid, vitamin B5. A biology professor at Mary Washington College in Virginia, Thomas L. Johnson, Ph.D., claims that daily supplements of pantothenic acid completely cleared age spots in just a few months. However, be careful when considering vitamin B5 supplements. These supplements can change the action of high blood-pressure and blood-thinning drugs. Pantothenic acid may also increase premature skin wrinkles in people who smoke. Pantothenic acid is found naturally in yeast, whole-grain products, liver, salmon, eggs, beans, seeds, peanuts, mushrooms, elderberries and citrus fruit. The best way to prevent age spots is by avoiding exposure to the sun and sunlamps.

• Rough skin on the feet can be a problem. For treatment, soak the feet once a day in warm water. Then gently use a pumice stone to rub away the rough calluses on the feet. Be careful with a pumice stone. You can rub away too much skin, causing bleeding and skin damage. If you soak and rub your feet daily for a couple of weeks, the rough spots should disappear without damaging the feet. Each day after using the pumice stone, apply a good moisturizer or petroleum jelly and cover your feet with socks. Sleeping in the socks will keep the moisturizer on your feet during the night.

• Sudden skin rash could be caused by exposure to high-intensity mercury lamps, according to the *Harvard Medical School Health Letter*. High-intensity lamps are usually covered by protective glass to block the ultraviolet rays. However, just a small hole in the protective glass can result in exposure to ultraviolet rays. The New Jersey Department of Health reported a case where 69 out of 89 girls on a school basketball team developed irritation of the eyes and skin rash. The outbreak was caused by a small hole in the protective coating of the mercury vapor light in the gym where the girls' team had just played.

• Photosensitivity is an exaggerated reaction to sunlight, which may be caused by using certain drugs, cosmetics, or perfumes, reports *Patient Care* (6:15). Photosensitivity is not a true allergic reaction, unless the reaction is extremely severe or unusual. Redness, swelling, hives and itching are symptoms of photosensitivity. If your skin is photosensitive, it reacts to the sun more quickly and more severely than normal. Some of the drugs that can lead to photosensitivity are thiazide diuretics, tetracycline, antidiabetics, psoralens, oral contraceptives, antipsychotics, antidepressants, antihistamines, antibacterials, anticancer drugs, and corticosteroids. Coal tar products, coal tar dyes, musk fragrance, some perfumes, and even some sunscreens can also cause photosensitivity.

A Nutritional Deficiency May Cause Acne

Anyone who has experienced even mild acne remembers well the forbidden foods: chocolate, sweets, soft drinks and greasy or fatty foods.

Although diet may play a minor role in the development of acne, research does not support the popular opinion that it is a major cause, according to *Nutrition Review*.

Rather than concentrating on removing things from the diet, perhaps the focus should center on what nutrients can be added.

While there is an overall clinical impression that a relationship between acne and sweet foods exists, some dermatologists attack such notions and claim the only unique thing about the supposed offending foods is they are "delicious and delectable for the adolescent palate," the article says.

Researchers have found that a diet low in zinc may worsen or activate acne. A study involving a group of teenage boys with severe acne discovered they had significantly lower serum zinc levels than normal. Patients treated with zinc supplements showed a marked improvement. The recommended daily dietary allowance of zinc is 15 mg. per day for adults.

Vitamin A has been used to treat acne for some time, and recent studies have confirmed its effectiveness. Acne sufferers have been found to have low levels of retinol-binding protein (RBP), which is closely related to vitamin A.

It is not known why acne patients have zinc and vitamin A deficiencies.

Too Much Washing Harms the Skin

What could be more harmless than the daily practice of washing your face?

Believe it or not, there are some hazards to that personal hygiene ritual, according to *Prevention* magazine.

Dr. Harvey Blank, heading an advisory panel to the Food and Drug Administration, studied the effects of deodorant soaps and plain soaps on human skin.

Other studies have revealed that antiseptics absorbed through the skin may interfere with bodily processes, retarding the growth of brain tissue in infants and interfering with the immune system, which fights infections and cancer.

Also, Blank notes that not all bacteria on the skin are harmful. Removing the harmless bacteria allows "harmful, disease-causing bacteria" to take their place, Blank says.

"Just killing bacteria does not necessarily mean you are doing good," he adds.

A Laundry Product
That Can Irritate
Your Skin

Skin irritation in the groin or vaginal area may be caused by your fabric softener! Itching in the pelvic area can be caused by fabric softener left on your underwear, explains Dr. Duane Townsend of the University of California/Davis Medical Center.

Tight underwear, especially synthetic materials that do not breathe, can cause rashes and skin irritation on their own, Townsend says. But adding a fabric softener can often make the problems worse. Townsend reports that any fabric softener can cause the problem. If you suffer from this type of skin irritation, eliminating fabric softener, wearing loose, cotton underwear, and using non-colored, non-scented toilet paper is recommended.

SMOKING

A New Reason To Quit

Smoking is harmful to your health, but is it damaging to your career as well? That's right, according to a recent survey.

Non-smokers have a better chance of making top management than smokers, based on the results of a survey by Robert Half International. The survey discovered that only 22 per cent of top executives smoked, while 30 per cent of middle management and 38 per cent of workers smoked.

As smoking continues to become less acceptable in the workplace, it seems that smokers will be seen as being less healthy and less acceptable in management positions.

Early Menopause?
It May Be Caused
By This Habit

Women smokers suffer many unique health problems including early menopause.

"Cigarette smoking has an anti-estrogen effect," *The Health Letter* says. Women smokers have their menopause an average of two years earlier than non-smokers. The decreased estrogen leads to osteoporosis and an increased risk of broken hips and collapsed vertebrae. The anti-estrogen effect of smoking is also believed responsible for the tendency of women smokers to lose their teeth prematurely.

"Cigarette smoking has a major effect on a woman's reproductive ability," *The Health Letter* reports. It reduces fertility, increases the risk of spontaneous abortion, and may increase the risk of a misplaced placenta which can lead to a miscarriage. Smoking cigarettes increases the risk of invasive cancer of the cervix as well.

"There are also studies that suggest there may be long- term effects on infants born to mothers who smoke cigarettes," *The Health Letter* adds.

On top of all that, lung cancer has now replaced breast cancer as the leading cause of cancer among women. As many as 80 percent of the heart attacks among heavy smokers are believed to be caused by smoking.

If for no other reason, women may want to quit smoking because of its effect on appearance. Prolonged cigarette smoking has been implicated in an increase in facial wrinkles, particularly crow's-feet around the corners of the eyes.

"It has been shown that women who smoke

257

cigarettes may look ten or more years older than women of the same age who do not smoke," *The Health Letter* says.

SNEEZING

Sneezing Can Cause Broken Bones

Seventh-century Italy was plagued by a mysterious disease in which a victim would sneeze several times and drop dead. In desperation, the Pope suggested a blessing be pronouned on anyone who sneezed. That practice has continued to this day; although a sneeze is no longer a sign of imminent death, we still respond with: "God Bless You."

A sternutatory reflex, or sneeze, usually occurs when the inside of the nose is irritated, the *Harvard Medical School Health Letter* says. Causes include viruses, allergies, or inhaling something like pepper. Looking at a bright light and withdrawal from narcotics also precipitate sneezing in some people.

Usually a sneeze is no more injurious than a yawn. However, a severe bout can cause nose bleeding. In some cases, cartilage in the nose or throat, or bones in the sinus or middle ear may break. Abdominal pressure that builds just before the sneeze may also aggravate hemorrhoids or hernias.

The best treatment for a sneeze is obviously to

remove or relieve the cause. For chronic sneezing many still place a finger under their nose and press against their upper teeth. Another method is supposedly more effective: press your finger hard against the glabella (the flat area between the eyebrows).

If all that fails, look on the bright side: at least you don't live in the seventh century.

STRESS

Relaxation Techniques
To Improve
Your Health

One of the best investments you can make in your health may be your easy chair, according to some medical experts. Relaxation, if practiced regularly, can lower blood pressure, reduce heart rate and alleviate many chronic pains.

Dr. Herbert Benson, author of the best seller, *The Relaxation Response,* and another book, *Beyond The Relaxation Response,* is a cardiologist and associate professor at Harvard Medical School. He, along with many other specialists, believes relaxation can relieve stress, tension and anxiety, which are major causes of heart attacks and strokes.

Worry, stress and tension activate the sympathetic nervous system, which releases the hormones adrenaline or noradrenaline into your body's system. During an emergency they help you to cope with the situation. However, emotional stresses can make this protective mechanism backfire, and instead of helping your nerves and muscles, the hormones tend to attack your own body's defenses.

Relaxing to cope with this emotional stress requires little time and no expense. Here's a beginner's guide to relaxation based on Dr. Benson's books:

• Sit or lie in a comfortable position. Make sure there are few distractions until you learn these techniques.

• Close your eyes.

• Take a deep breath slowly. Let it out slowly. Think about how the air feels entering and leaving your body, as you inhale and exhale.

• Consciously relax your muscles. If it helps, start with your toes and tell each section of your body to relax. For example, say to yourself, "Toes on my right foot relax. Now, toes on my left foot relax." Continue until you reach the top of your head.

• Concentrate on only one thought or word. This helps to clear your mind of random thoughts. For example say the word "Peace," or even the simple prayer "My peace I give unto you" (John 14:27), and repeat it over and over. Adopt a passive attitude toward intrusive thoughts, letting them enter, but then letting them go. Continue repeating your word or phrase.

At first, relax for only five or ten minutes.

Gradually build the length of your sessions to 15 or 20 minutes. Taking a bath after work or before bedtime is an excellent way to use your relaxation techniques. Dr. Benson recommends two short sessions daily to relax you.

After you finish your session, sit quietly for a moment or two, then let regular thoughts back into your consciousness. Open your eyes and sit quietly another moment or two. Don't try to get up too quickly.

You can also learn to relax during aerobic exercises like walking, jogging and swimming. First warm up with stretches and deep breathing.

Then, if you are walking, concentrate on the rhythm of your steps. Say to yourself, "Right one, left one. Right two, left two," and so forth. If you are jogging concentrate on your breathing. Count as you inhale and exhale, "Breathe in—one, breathe out—one. Breathe in—two, breathe out—two." If you are lounging at the pool or at the beach, repeat your chosen word or phrase.

Of course you should always consult your physician when treating pain or physical symptoms of illness which persistently cause discomfort. Dr. Benson advises the combination of proven medical therapies with your own relaxation routine for optimal health and well-being.

Dream Away Bad Feelings

Dreams play a larger role in our mental and physical health than was once believed. When we dream, we're sorting out our emotions and eliminating stress from our systems. This helps to restore nerves, muscles, and vital organs to use while we're awake.

Nobel prize winner, Dr. Francis Crick of the Salk Institute and his colleague, British biologist Dr. Graeme Mitchison, explained the results of their dream research as reported in a recent *Atlanta Journal and Constitution* newspaper article.

They claim, "We dream in order to forget." Dreams are our way of disposing of hundreds of random thoughts and associations our senses pick up daily. Like garbage trucks, dreams cart off the unwanted or unimportant information we've accumulated, relieving tension and stress. As these random thoughts and bits of information are released, the higher brain weaves them into patterns, which accounts for many strange and unusual stories people link to their dreams.

Other research shows a person deprived of sleep will increase dreaming when given the first opportunity of undisturbed sleep. Releasing this over-abundance of sensations accumulated during sleep deprivation allows the body to restore its emotional balance.

Therefore, it is the process of dreaming that helps promote good mental and physical health, not the content of our dreams. Dreaming allows us to release tension and stress, so that during our deeper stages of sleep our bodies can restore the physical resources needed to cope with the next day's activities.

A Simple Therapy
for Stress

Just thinking about a chocolate sundae can reduce your stress, researchers from Yale University report. In the study, stress levels were reduced when people were asked to imagine eating their favorite food.

Tests also showed that smelling favorite food fragrances, perhaps chocolate chip cookies just the way mom used to make them, helped people relax as much as standard relaxation therapy, according to Michael Yapko of the Milton Erickson Institute in San Diego. People learning to relax by visualizing their favorite peaceful places and times should also try visualizing eating their favorite foods.

Doctors warn, however, that this technique should not be used by people with eating disorders or weight problems.

STROKES

A Common Medication That May Help

An ingredient in common cough syrups and cold medicine may help reduce the crippling effects of strokes, a study at Stanford University in California discovered. Dextromethorphan seems to help the brain survive when it is deprived of oxygen during a stroke.

The research is still preliminary, so the researchers are not suggesting taking cough syrup for stroke prevention or healing.

Is Snoring Related to Strokes?

People who snore disturb the sleep of anyone within hearing distance. Now there is some disturbing news for snorers themselves: their nocturnal noises indicate an increased risk of stroke.

In a comparison between 177 stroke patients and 177 stroke-free men at the University of Helsinki, Finland, snoring was found to be "more than twice as common in the stroke patients," the researchers said (*Medical Tribune*).

These people who snored reported snoring

always or often, while the non-snorer group consisted of people who snored occasionally or never.

Although "habitual snoring has been associated with arterial hypertension," Dr. Heikk Palomaki, a neurologist at the University of Helsinki, says, "we really don't know what mechanism may be at work here."

In both groups risk factors such as "hypertension, diabetes mellitus, smoking and alcohol consumption" were considered, but it was snoring which clearly stood out as the greatest risk factor for stroke, the *Medical Tribune* reports.

A New Way To Detect Blocked Arteries

A new test spots clogged arteries without X-rays or injections and could prevent strokes. Developed at Imperial College in London, the new procedure uses ultrasound to identify arteries blocked as little as 15 percent. Until now, ultrasound testing could only identify blockages of 50 percent or more and those blocks were already life-threatening.

A sensor about the size of a small flashlight is held up to the patient's cartoid artery in the neck. In about ten minutes, the sensor allows the non-irritating ultrasound waves to be read and analyzed for blockages by a physician using computerized instrumentation. Ultrasound is completely harmless to the patient and doesn't have any side effects.

Doctors are pleased with this new technology because it will help screen healthy patients, as well as high-risk patients. Early screening for blocked arteries can lead to better care and prevention, says Dr. Richard Kitney, who directed the research at Imperial College.

TATTOOS

A New Way to Remove Them

Lasers can remove tattoos with better results and lower infection rates than traditional removal methods.

For years, people with tattoos that were once treasured but now unwanted have sought a way to have them removed. Many things affect the success of laser removal, like how old the tattoo is, what kind of dye and techniques were used, and the colors involved. However, Dr. Javier Ruiz Esparza at the University of California, San Diego School of Medicine says that laser removal is now the preferred method of removal. The laser technique leaves less scar tissue, is less painful, and has a lower infection rate, reports Esparza.

TOOTH DECAY

Something You Should Know About Taking Antihistamines

Did you know that if you are taking antihistamines you have more risk of tooth decay?

Antihistamines dry up the saliva in the mouth and nasal passages. The decrease in saliva can cause an increase in the number of cavities and gum problems, according to an article in *Family Circle*.

If you take antihistamines for your allergies, brush your teeth more often and drink more water or other sugar-free drinks to avoid an increase in dental problems.

TOOTHACHE

Tips To Relieve The Pain

You've developed a toothache, and while you are waiting to see your dentist you decide to lie down for awhile.

That's the wrong thing to do, says Dr. Stephen Schwartz of the American Association of Endodontists. Schwartz suggests sitting up with a toothache because it lowers the blood pressure in the head and lessens the pain of the toothache!

Swallowing an over-the-counter painkiller like aspirin, ibuprofen or acetaminophen will also help. And the American Dental Association suggests swishing warm water in your mouth for immediate relief when you have a toothache. Be sure to contact your dentist as soon as possible.

TOXIC-SHOCK SYNDROME

What Tampon Packages Don't Tell You Can Be Fatal

A new study at the Center for Disease Control (CDC) in Atlanta offers evidence that toxic-shock syndrome is more common in those who use high-absorbency tampons, *Prevention* magazine reports.

The CDC says the major risk of potentially fatal toxic-shock syndrome is tampon use. The greater the absorbency of a tampon, the greater the risk.

Inserts in tampon packages advise using the least absorbent variety but don't say why. The study by the CDC says, "the risk of toxic-shock increases 37 percent for each gram increase in tampon absorbency."

Claire Broome, M.D., coauthor of the CDC study, says products don't give adequate information; therefore, choosing the best one is difficult. Until the Food and Drug Administration requires that information be listed on the box, use the least absorbent tampon possible, Broome advises.

If during your menstrual period you develop a

high fever, rash, vomiting or diarrhea, discontinue the use of the tampon you are wearing and see a doctor immediately.

ULCERS

Home Treatment For Ulcers in Sight

There is a pessimistic saying among ulcer researchers: "Once an ulcer always an ulcer."

Although drugs, both prescription and over-the-counter, have been found to effectively treat ulcers, 75 to 90 percent of ulcer patients have flare-ups again, according to *Prevention* magazine.

The findings of two Australian doctors may now change all that.

Robin Warren, a pathologist, and Barry Marshall, a gastroenterologist at the Royal Peth Hospital, discovered after hundreds of tests that an unusual bacterium was present in most cases of duodenal ulcer (the most common form of ulcer), *Prevention* reports. They also discovered that a bismuth compound cleared up the bacteria and the ulcers. (Bismuth had been used to treat bacterial infections like syphilis in the 1940's, prior to the discovery of penicillin). A bismuth compound is the primary ingredient in Pepto Bismol®.

In their latest test "30 percent of ulcer patients who took the bismuth compound alone were clear of the bacterium, compared to none in the group given the usual ulcer treatment . . . Tagamet,"

Prevention reports.

Seventy-five percent of those who took an antibacterial drug along with the bismuth compound were completely free of the bacterium and the ulcer.

As *Prevention* points out, "the real test for any ulcer treatment is the relapse rate." On that score only 30 percent of the patients who received both bismuth and the antibiotic had a relapse, compared with between 80 and 100 percent of the Tagamet patients.

The two doctors believe that the bacterium they identified somehow damages the "cling-wrap-like" lining of the stomach, as Dr. Marshall puts it, which allows stomach acid to eat a hole in the lining, causing an ulcer.

The doctors claim the antibiotic and bismuth compound treatment has a 75 percent success rate in curing an ulcer permanently. A two-week therapy session using the two medicines costs only $30. And bismuth is easily and inexpensively available in Pepto Bismol.

Prevention stresses that these studies are still "preliminary," but the medical community is encouraged and interested. So too are ulcer sufferers.

Balloon Stops Ulcer Bleeding

Techniques for stopping a bleeding ulcer have met with mixed success in the past. According to *Medical World News*, bleeding ulcer sufferers have a 10 percent mortality rate partially due to the inadequacy of present blood staunching techniques.

Dr. T. Vincent Taylor, of the University of Manchester, England, found that "inflating a balloon in the duodenum (the first and widest part of the small intestine) is the quickest, easiest, and least expensive way to staunch ulcer bleeding."

Testing his new device with animals and two patients, Taylor found that the "hemorrhage stopped immediately when the balloon was inflated," according to *Medical World News*.

The balloon is fitted over the end of a small tube called an endoscope and introduced into the duodenal cap during examination for upper gastrointestinal hemorrhage. The balloon is then inflated by an attached tube. When the balloon is inflated the endcoscope is taken out. The balloon can be deflated and removed easily once the bleeding has stopped.

In each patient the balloon was left in overnight and then removed. Bleeding did not resume except minimally in one patient four days later, the article

277

reports.

The balloon conforms to the contours of the duodenal cap when inserted, and the shape of the duodenum prevents the balloon from slipping out when the endoscope is removed.

A Common Habit That May Cause Ulcers

If the first thing you want in the morning is a cup of coffee, you may be increasing your chances of getting an ulcer.

Drinking coffee on an empty stomach may cause an ulcer, warns Dr. Robert Davis of the Digestive Disease Laboratory in Houston. It is important to note that both caffeinated and decaffeinated coffee increase acid production in your stomach and, thus, can cause ulcers, especially if taken alone, says Dr. Davis.

WEIGHT LOSS

Have You Thought Of It This Way?

You've tried to convince yourself in all kinds of ways that you want to stick to your diet. But have you ever let your money do the talking?

Dr. Arnold Andersen, Director of the Eating and Weight Disorders Clinic in Baltimore, suggests thinking of your diet like an annual expense. Rather than paying $500 for rent each month you could reduce your rent to $400. Over the year you would save a lot of money. If you can compare your rent to your diet, you can see that just cutting back a little can make a healthy difference over a long period of time. Reducing the amount of high-calorie and high-fat foods you eat even by 10 percent, will help you lose weight and improve your overall health.

Some Common Misconceptions

You probably know a lot about how to lose weight, but some of what you "know" may not be "so." Here are three common misconceptions.

Exercise is important for weight loss and overall health, but not all exercise will help you lose weight. Recent studies by Dr. Gran Gwinup of the University of California Medical Center show that swimming actually increases body weight. Dr. Gwinup says that since swimming is an aerobic exercise it is excellent for the heart, but it increases the muscle bulk and doesn't contribute to a weight loss program.

Using artificial sweeteners does not guarantee weight loss, reports a new study by the American Cancer Society. In a study of 78,000 dieters, people using artificial sweeteners gained more weight than people not using substitutes. The artificial sweeteners did not cause the weight gain. However, the researchers concluded that the people thought they were cutting back by using the artificial sweeteners, and they just didn't limit their calories overall. Don't be lulled into a false sense of security — reducing total caloric intake and exercising are the only true ways to lose weight.

Avoid diet pills, even prescription drugs, unless your doctor believes they are absolutely necessary. Recently a 37-year-old woman nearly died when her heart stopped, Dr. Harry R. Gibbs reports in the *New England Journal of Medicine* (318:17,1127). The woman had been taking three drugs prescribed for weight loss—phentermine hydrochloride, thyroid, and trichlormethiazide—and didn't have any heart or artery problems. Gibbs warns that using inappropriate prescription drugs to treat obesity, even in someone without heart problems, can lead to "sudden catastrophic events."

When You Eat, Not How Much, Can Peel Off Pounds

There's an old dieting maxim: "Eat breakfast like a king, lunch like a prince, and dinner like a pauper."

Is it really true that eating more in the morning than in the evening makes a difference in how much weight you lose?

Yes, according to a study reported in the *Journal of the American Medical Association* (JAMA).

In a study at the National Institute of Health in Bethesda, Maryland, three patients were fed a 400-calorie meal once a day for 10 day periods. They would eat either a breakfast at 8 a.m or a dinner at 5 p.m each period. The study was then repeated with each patient.

Two of the patients "had notably greater weight loss," JAMA says, when they ate in the morning instead of in the evening. The researchers concluded that weight loss was greatly affected by the "timing of the food intake," JAMA reports.

It appears that only breakfast should indeed be the king of meals.

An Unusual Twist

Being fat can save your life! Dr. Kenneth Warner has discovered that fewer overweight people die violently than thin people.

This seems like an ironic discovery since being overweight can cause an early death due to health problems. But Dr. Warner, a medical examiner in Alabama, found that although one of every four people is overweight, among those who died violently, only one person in eight was overweight. He speculates that overweight people live a more sedentary lifestyle so they aren't as likely to suffer a violent death. For example, they aren't participating in dangerous sports like hang-gliding.

People who weighed more than 10 percent over their ideal body weight were classified as overweight in this study.

WRINKLES

A Cream That Makes Your Skin
Look Years Younger

You've enjoyed all those years of being in the sun, and now your skin has to pay for it, right? Maybe not.

Now there's a cream available that is medically proven to "de-age" skin. The cream is the prescription drug Retin-A®, which has been sold as an anti-acne product since 1971. But the users discovered smoother, less wrinkled skin was a side effect of Retin-A®, and now scientific studies have proven it. Researchers at the University of Michigan found Retin-A® (chemical name— tretinoin) repairs the damage that sun does to your skin. It cannot fix sagging skin or deep wrinkles but it does increase the depth of the skin and helps skin look and feel smoother, reports the *Journal of the American Medical Association* (JAMA 259:4,527). Plus, the report says that Retin-A® caused a "disappearance of the cellular abnormalities known to be forerunners of cancer."

People taking Retin-A® should apply it at night, then use a sunscreen (SPF at least 15) during the day since the skin becomes very sensitive during the restoration. Retin-A® is a derivative of vitamin A but taking vitamin A or using a vitamin A cream will *not* give you the same effect. Retin-A® is available only by prescription in cream, gel or liquid forms and costs about $20.00 for a three month supply.

Concluding Remarks

The natural healing secrets in this book are based on medical reports, but don't overlook the supernatural healing power of God. God is our Creator and the Master Physician. If you put your faith and trust in God, by following Jesus Christ, your prayers for healing will be answered according to God's will.

If you would like to know more about how to know God and have eternal life through a personal relationship with Jesus Christ, please write to FC&A, Dept JC 88, 103 Clover Green, Peachtree City, Georgia, 30269. We believe getting to know God better will change your life!

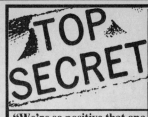

"DO YOU KNOW THESE NATURAL HEALTH SECRETS AND CURES?"

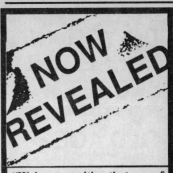

NOW REVEALED

"We're so positive that one of our health tips or cures will work for you that we'll send you a free gift just for trying them."

By Frank K. Wood)

FC&A, a Peachtree City, Georgia, health publisher, announced today the release of a new book for the general public, *"Encyclopedia of Natural Health Secrets and Cures"*.

LOOK AT THESE LIFE AND HEALTH SAVING SECRETS \REVEALED IN THIS NEW BOOK

- Senility doesn't have to happen! This pleasant remedy does wonders to help people think and feel young.
- Cancer from your electric wires? Don't laugh.
- Alzheimer's Disease. Something to avoid that may cause it.
- Sexual activity and memory loss. What's the connection?
- Stop dieting! Easy way to lose weight.
- Avoid arthritis symptoms. Do this.
- Warm in the winter? Try this.

- Zap a cold. Suck on this (it's not what you think).
- Hair loss in women. How you can often stop it.
- Wrinkle reduction: tips from an expert.
- Cancer from your basement? Check this.
- Low I.Q.? It may be the way you sleep.
- A dramatic new way to avoid allergies.
- How tomatoes can help prevent this bowel problem.
- Asthma? Stop doing this and avoid attacks.
- Incontinence: this helps.
- This mineral lowers blood pressure.
- Bronchitis: the chief, easily prevented cause.
- The water you drink may keep you from getting cancer.
- This kind of apple a day won't keep the doctor away.
- Help avoid breast cancer.

- A laxative that causes cancer.